THE 7-DAY BONE BROTH DIET PLAN & COOKBOOK

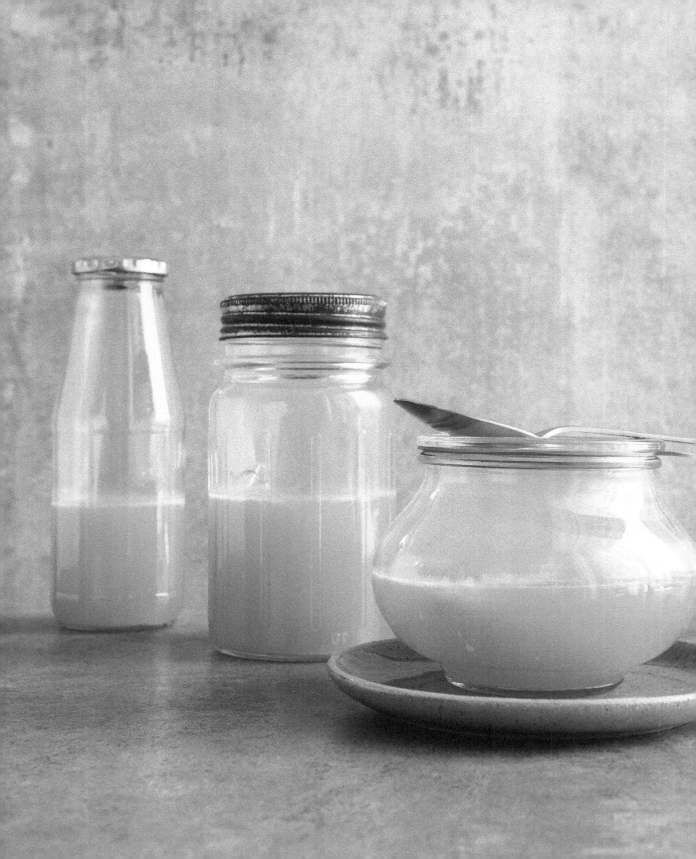

THE
7-DAY BONE BROTH DIET PLAN & COOKBOOK

HEALING BONE BROTH RECIPES TO BOOST HEALTH AND PROMOTE WEIGHT LOSS

Meredith Cochran

Foreword by Thomas Cowan, MD

ROCKRIDGE
PRESS

Photography © Nadine Greeff/Stocksy, cover, pp. ii-iii, vi, 138 & back cover; Michael Wissing/Stockfood, p. 2; Shea Evans/Stockfood, p. 10; Wolfgang Schardt/Jalag/Stockfood, pp. 18 & 66; Gräfe & Unzer Verlag/Kramp + Gölling/Stockfood, pp. 28 & 54; Maya Visnyei/Stockfood, p. 40; Gräfe & Unzer Verlag/Kramp + Gölling/Stockfood, p. 54; Justina Ramanauskiene/Stockfood, p. 60; Ian Wallace/Stockfood, p. 74; Tom Swalens/PhotoCuisine/Stockfood, p. 96; Jan-Peter Westermann /Zabert Sandmann Verlag/Stockfood, p. 108; Jonathan Gregson/Stockfood, p. 116; B.&.E. Dudzinski/Stockfood, p. 130.

Author photo courtesy of Meredith Cochran

ISBN: Print 978-1-62315-998-6 | eBook 978-1-62315-999-3

*To Jazz: for your unrelenting
ability to make me laugh*

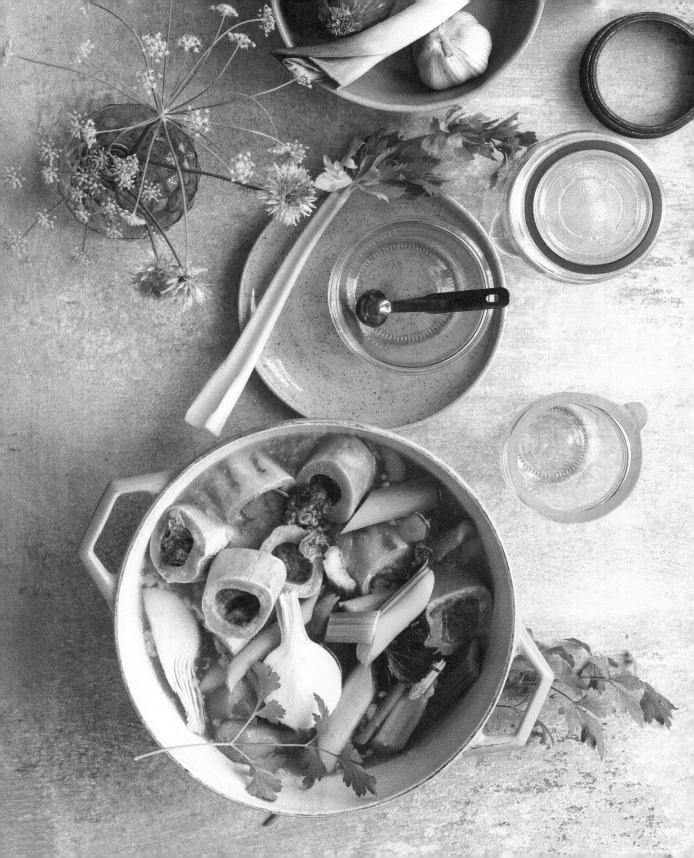

CONTENTS

FOREWORD

A few years ago, I saw an interview with Kobe Bryant in which he was asked to reveal the secrets of how he remains so strong and fit in spite of his "advanced age" (for a professional basketball player). While his answer included the usual tributes to hard work and dedication, he also said a big part of the reason was his daily consumption of bone broth. It was then that I realized bone broth had entered mainstream American culture.

I first got involved with making and consuming bone broth through my friend and coauthor Sally Fallon in the mid-1990s. During that time, bones from pastured animals were hard to come by and virtually none of my patients knew what I was talking about when I mentioned it. It's incredible that just twenty years later, the availability of good bone broth and the knowledge of the benefits of bone broth to our health have become commonplace. *The 7-Day Bone Broth Diet Plan & Cookbook* pushes us even further down the road of understanding the rationale behind the consumption of daily bone broth. It also helps that Meredith runs one of the best manufacturers of bone broth out there, Osso Good. Personally, I am both a regular maker of bone broth and a consumer of Osso Good bone broths.

My favorite part of *The 7-Day Bone Broth Diet Plan & Cookbook*, besides the wonderful recipes and illuminating information, is the innovative and practical suggestion to do a 7-day bone broth "cleanse" as a way of introducing the consumption of bone broth into your diet as you embark on the path to improving your health. This cleanse is not only easy and satisfying but, as Meredith suggests, it will aid in your quest to improve your health—no matter what your current health status is. The bone broth cleanse works from the inside out, addressing our important gut health first, and setting the stage for further healing down the road.

This innovative approach to introducing people to the magic of bone broth, written by an expert in the art and science of it, will be a valuable addition to your library and to your life.

Thomas Cowan, MD
Author of *Human Heart, Cosmic Heart* **and** *The Fourfold Path to Healing*

INTRODUCTION

Congratulations! You have decided to take control of your health through one of the most nutrient-dense foods available: bone broth. For those of you new to bone broth, it is a savory, water-based liquid in which bones are simmered. This prehistoric food was an important staple in our ancestors' diets because it contained nutrients not found in lean cuts of meat. Because we can't consume bones directly, we must slowly simmer them over long periods of time to draw out liquid that nourishes our bodies with nutrients. Today, you can purchase high-quality bone broth or make your own bone broth slowly simmered at home to regain your ancestral heritage.

I first heard of bone broth while I was studying to become an acupuncturist and herbalist at the American College of Traditional Chinese Medicine. I was with a group of friends when I heard a few of them discussing how much they loved bone broth and how hard it was to find a good source for it. One of them told us how awesome it was after a long bike ride. It left him feeling reenergized and soothed aching joints. Later that week, my professor told us that it is an excellent vehicle for Chinese herbs. As a student in desperate need of nourishing food on the go, I headed straight for the kitchen to make my own. After a few failed attempts, I was able to make bone broth that I was proud of. Years and many recipes later, I cofounded the all-natural bone broth company, Osso Good.

The 7-Day Bone Broth Diet Plan & Cookbook isn't just a "diet" that you will do for a week and then give up on. Rather, this book will give you the tools necessary to make bone broth at home, implement easy tweaks to your routine and to incorporate bone broths into your daily life. It is also important to note that this book focuses on healing your body from the inside out, and while this often leads to weight loss, that is not the goal. You should never feel hungry when eating from the diet portion of the book. The point isn't to starve your body of the nutrients it needs, but rather to flood your system with the most nutrient-dense foods available. While this may seem counterintuitive, think of a well-oiled machine. It, too, runs smoothly when given plenty of high-quality oil and fuel so it can perform the simplest or most complex task.

We are going to start by going over the basics of bone broth, how to make your own, and how to stick to the bone broth diet in part 1. Part 2 consists of my favorite bone broth recipes for everything from drinks and sides to stews and entrées. I am so excited to share my bone broth knowledge with you!

Meredith Cochran

Part One

Bone Broth for Better Health

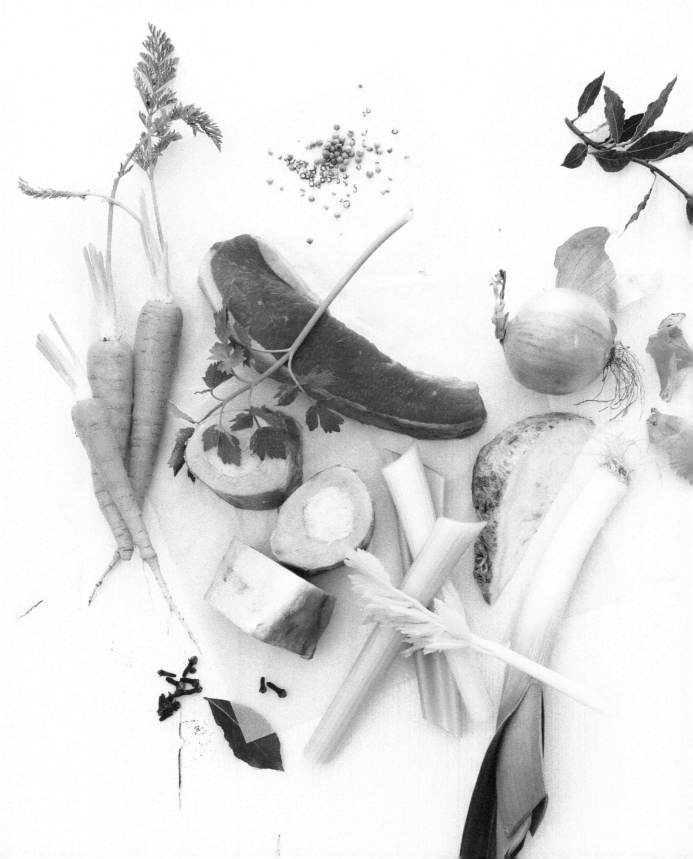

CHAPTER ONE

bone broth diet basics

The 7-Day Bone Broth Diet Plan & Cookbook is all about rebooting your gut and setting you on a path to a better-feeling you with better eating habits. The main idea of this book is simple: consume 40 ounces of bone broth per day plus whole foods as needed to improve your path to better gut health. This means eating only pastured and grassfed proteins, good saturated fats (like avocado, coconut oil, and ghee), and organic vegetables. Avoid dairy, grains, and sugar because they cause inflammation in your gut. Bone broth is naturally anti-inflammatory and improves digestion, allowing your gut to do a mini "reset." In this chapter, we are going to go over everything you need to know about bone broth. Let's begin!

Why Bone Broth?

There is a reason why your grandma always cooked up a pot of chicken soup when you were feeling ill. For centuries, bone broth has been used by grandmothers and prescribed by physicians to help heal you from the inside out. By slowly simmering the bones, meat, tendons, ligaments, and feet of an animal, you are able to transfer their nourishing benefits into an easily digestible liquid combination of gelatin, essential amino acids, and minerals. Fans of bone broth say it:

- Supports the immune system
- Promotes healthy digestion by healing and sealing the gut
- Strengthens bones, skin, nails, and hair
- Reduces inflammation and joint pain
- Boosts energy levels
- Promotes better sleep

Bone broth is rich, satisfying, nutrient dense, and has the ability to fill your belly without adding many calories. It is known for its ability to detoxify your liver and help rid your entire body of toxins. It simultaneously adds collagen to your skin, allowing your face to stay youthful. Most importantly, bone broth heals and seals your gut. Did you know that the surface area of your gut is 30 to 40 square meters (322 to 430 square feet)? Every system in your body is connected and at the center of it all is your gut. With about 70 percent of the immune system located in the gut, poor gut health is linked to hormone imbalance, eczema and other skin-related diseases, autoimmune diseases (including arthritis), anxiety, depression, chronic fatigue, and diabetes, to name a few. Bone broth increases absorption of nutrients while also creating the perfect environment for your gut flora (the bacteria in your gut offering a mutualistic relationship and having the ability to change based on diet). Because bone broth is naturally anti-inflammatory, with regular consumption you might also shed weight. Let's learn more about it.

The 7-Day Bone Broth Diet

We wanted to create a weeklong diet that would give you the tools required to reset your gut and to experience a better-feeling you. By flooding your system with the most nutrient-dense foods available, you should not feel hungry on this cleanse. At about 12 grams of protein per 8-ounce serving, you'll be amazed at how full you feel after your 40 ounces of daily bone broth. You'll be able to eat a ton of delicious food during the week. Let's go over what you can and can't consume.

WHAT YOU CAN EAT:

- Bone broth that must be thick and gelatinous for healing benefits
- All meat that is responsibly raised, including chicken, beef, pork, lamb, turkey, bison, and wild-caught fish
- Eggs from pasture-raised hens
- Ghee, coconut oil, olive oil, avocados, sprouted nuts, and sprouted beans
- All organic fruits, including but not limited to apples, bananas, blackberries, blueberries, cantaloupe, cherries, grapes, kiwi, lemons, limes, all melons, oranges, peaches, pears, pineapple, and strawberries
- All organic vegetables, including but not limited to arugula, beets, bell peppers, bok choy, broccoli, Brussels sprouts, cabbage, celery, carrots, cucumbers, garlic, jalapeños, kale, leeks, mushrooms, onions, parsnips, peas, plantains, romaine, spinach, sprouts, squash, sweet potatoes, tomatoes, and zucchini
- All organic herbs, including but not limited to basil, bay leaves, cilantro, mint, sage, and thyme

WHAT YOU CAN'T EAT:

- All dairy, including butter, milk, and yogurt, with the exception of ghee
- All processed sugars and artificial sugars, including all foods containing them such as soda and prepackaged meals
- All wheat and grains, including bread and quinoa
- Processed meats or lunch meats containing gluten, nitrites, or sweeteners
- Corn, rice, and white potatoes
- All oils except olive oil
- Alcohol

The Benefits of the 7-Day Bone Broth Diet

At this point, you may be asking yourself, "Why should I do this?" The better question is, "Why shouldn't I do this?" This diet gives you the freedom to eat until you're full and still feel amazing! A Harvard study published in the medical journal *Nature* found significant changes in the makeup of the gut bacteria occurring just three days after a dietary change. Did you know that your gut is known as the second brain? And that the enteric cells that make up your gut consist of more than 100 million neurons? That's more than your spinal cord. You can also find a wealth of neurotransmitters, immune cells, and endorphins. By healing your gut, you are also healing your immune system and improving your mood. The 7-day bone broth diet is perfect because you can flood your system with as much nourishing food as you want, along with 40 ounces of bone broth a day. There are so many benefits. Here is a short list:

- Eating real food until full and still losing weight
- Strengthened hair, skin, and nails
- Improved joint health
- Deeper, sounder sleep
- A more habitable environment for your gut flora
- Boosted immune system
- Decreased inflammation
- Feeling more focused
- Improved digestion
- Increased energy
- Feeling more comfortable in your body, which radiates to those around you

A Superfood Powerhouse

Today, traditional foods like bone broth are making a comeback. Let's be honest, we all want the nourishment that these foods bring. The gut has more nerve endings than the spine and manufactures more neurotransmitters than the brain. It is also the source of 95 percent of serotonin production. With insufficient serotonin, we are more likely to experience insomnia, depression, and other mood disorders. Let's take a closer look at what makes bone broth a superfood.

Glycosaminoglycans (GAGs)

Glycosaminoglycans are essential molecules in the body. Their primary role is to maintain and support collagen, elastin, and "bounce" between cells. They serve an integral role in connective tissues like tendons and cartilage. Some of the most important glycosaminoglycans include chondroitin sulfate, dermatan sulfate, keratan sulfate, and hyaluronate. Without GAGs, many people suffer from conditions such as autoimmunity, arthritis, leaky gut, Crohn's disease, irritable bowel syndrome, asthma, Alzheimer's disease, osteoarthritis, and acid reflux. Bone broth is rich in GAGs when you use the whole animal, including their joints.

Bone Marrow

Bone marrow is soft, gelatinous tissue in the middle of long bones. It is a potent source of both mesenchymal and hematopoietic stem cells, which together produce fat, cartilage, bone, and blood cells. Stem cells are incredibly important for your body because they have the ability to constantly and rapidly produce new cells. These new cells are responsible for the creation of cartilage, bone, fat, muscle, lymph, and blood tissue. Bone marrow also plays a large role in immune function. Bone broth is rich in bone marrow when made properly with the long bones of the animal.

Collagen and Gelatin

The word "collagen" comes from the Greek word for glue. When made properly, you turn skin, cartilage, tendons, and ligaments into a gelatin-rich liquid glue. The cooking process of making broth breaks down the collagen proteins into gelatin, which provides the amino acids the body uses to make connective tissue. There are 29 types of collagen in the body, which comprise about 30 percent of the body's total protein. This tissue functions by strengthening the tendons that connect muscle to bone and ligaments that connect bone to bone. Collagen also supports the skin, which is the largest organ. Not only does collagen boost youthful firmness and elasticity, it also builds a barrier to prevent the absorption and possible spread of pathogens, toxins, microorganisms, and cancerous cells. The cornea and eye are supported by collagen, along with the placenta during pregnancy. It also gives strength to arteries, capillaries, and organs while keeping them supple. As we age, collagen production decreases, making it even more necessary to consume bone broth regularly.

Gelatin has been proven effective at increasing the digestibility of beans, wheat, oats, milk, and meat, and has been used for over a century in the treatment of malnourishment. In 1909, L. E. Hogan wrote, "[Gelatin in bone broth] is said to be retained by the most sensitive stomach and will nourish when almost nothing else will be tolerated." It has been proven effective in those with IBS, arthritis, leaky gut, and celiac disease. A good indicator of a high-quality bone broth is its Jell-O–like consistency, which is an indication of the amount of gelatin present. I will dive into this more in the recipes section.

Amino Acids

Bone broth is rich in amino acids such as proline and glycine, which are not available in lean cuts of meat. Proline, glycine, and glutamine are great for boosting your immune system, improving digestion, maintaining a balanced nervous system, and helping with muscle repair and growth.

Glycine is known as the anti-aging amino acid, and it contains the building blocks to create many other amino acids. This amino acid is essential because it maintains lean muscle, prevents loss of cartilage, reduces inflammation, aids in detoxification, improves energy, and helps maintain focus. The body needs plenty of glycine in order to fulfill many important functions. Proline is important for tissue repair, collagen formation, and blood pressure maintenance.

Glucosamine—which is formed when glutamine and glucose combine—is best known as a supplement that helps repair cartilage, decrease inflammation, alleviate joint pain, and increase range of motion. In the gut, glucosamine helps repair the defensive barrier in the mucosa.

Why Is Inflammation Important?

Inflammation is a normal response of your body to harmful stimuli. A few things that can cause inflammation are pathogens, trauma, toxins, alcohol, and stress. It's true; chronic stress can cause chronic inflammation, which in turn causes you to gain weight. This often leads to metabolic syndrome and cardiovascular disease with insulin resistance. By consuming foods that are anti-inflammatory, you can reverse this inflammation with time. The amount of time varies from person to person, but many have noticed a positive shift after successful completion of this diet.

Glutamine is known for its direct immune support, liver support for detoxification, and ability to boost metabolism. Glutamine is a vital amino acid in the 7-day bone broth diet for its ability to not only boost metabolism, but also to decrease cravings for sugar and other carbohydrates.

Minerals

Minerals such as calcium, magnesium, and potassium can all be found in high-quality bone broth. Calcium is an electrolyte vital to bone synthesis, nerve conduction, and muscle contraction. Soups containing vegetables, meat, and high-quality bone broth are an excellent source of dietary calcium. Magnesium is required in every cell that must use ATP (energy). Low magnesium is associated with neuromuscular, cardiovascular, and metabolic dysfunction including diabetes and hypertension. Potassium is essential for all nerve transmissions. Any deficiencies are associated with abnormal heart rhythm and cardiac function. A big bowl of bone broth soup containing meat and leafy greens is an excellent source of all three minerals.

Cartilage

The easiest way to understand what cartilage is would be to grab your ear and bend it. It's what gives your ear the ability to have shape and structure while still being flexible. Cartilage is incredibly resilient and is often attached to the ends of bones or used to hold tubes open. There are three different types of cartilage—hyaline, elastic, and fibrous—and they are composed of varying amounts of collagen and proteoglycans. Unlike most tissue, cartilage does not have a blood supply or nerve endings. As traditional Chinese medical doctors have known all along, cartilage-rich bone broth can in fact supply your body with the tools necessary to keep cartilage healthy and plentiful.

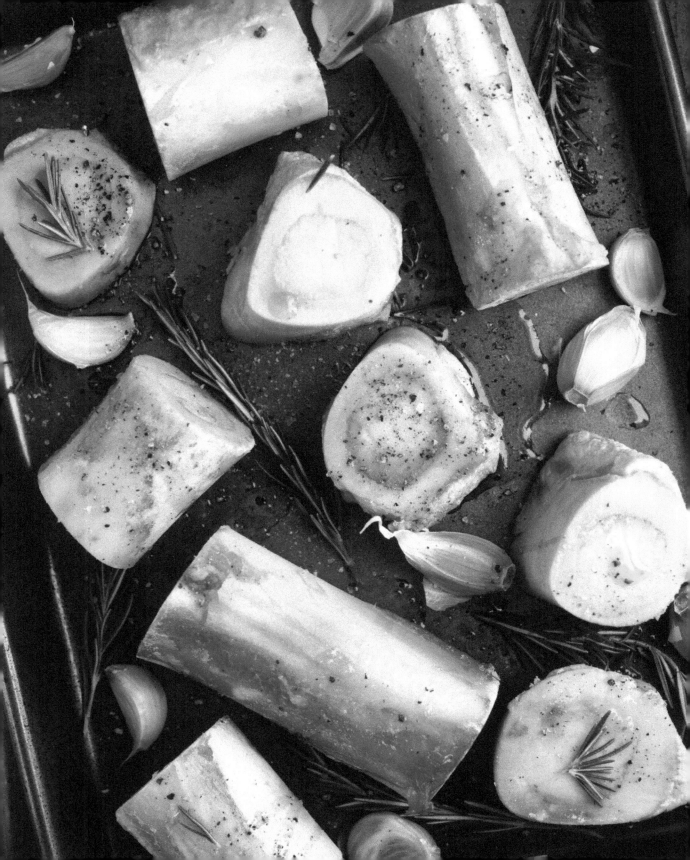

CHAPTER TWO

making homemade bone broth

Making homemade bone broth is a process, but with a little time and effort, even the most inexperienced chef can do it well. Remember to leave it alone once it begins cooking. Give yourself plenty of space and time to properly strain and cool your broth. And the most important part of making bone broth is sourcing the right ingredients.

The Best Bones

Bone broth is best when it's made with a lot of bones and meat. Because you are simmering them down a great deal to extract the minerals and amino acids, where you source your bones is incredibly important! If you use conventionally raised animals, you will also be consuming any antibiotics, hormones, pesticides, and toxins present. Aim to buy American Grassfed Association certified beef. These cattle are raised in the best conditions—they roam free and eat grass their whole lives—that go above and beyond organic standards. Cows that are grassfed but not grass finished are often given "fillers" of soy and corn at the end of their lives in an effort to plump them up for more meat. Chicken and turkey should be pasture raised. This gives the birds access to more than 100 square feet per bird to forage, and requires that they have full body access to the outdoors as well as shelter indoors, but no cages. Organic certifications give no requirements for quality of life, but rather only require that what the chickens consume must be organic. If unable to source pastured, grassfed, or grass finished, sourcing all organic ingredients is necessary.

You also want to use as many types of bones possible. By using some long bones, you get the bone marrow. The knuckles are perfect for cartilage. The neck bones are full of connective tissue. By using all three bone types, you're getting the most nutrient-dense bone broth possible.

Roasting Bones

The flavor of bone broth varies depending on the chef. All of my favorite recipes use roasted meat and bones. Roasting the bones gives the bone broth a richness that can't be replaced. It is important not to burn or overcook meat or bones because that flavor will impact your broth. Generally, you can roast bones at 375°F for about 15 minutes in your oven, but check the recipes section for specific cooking times and temperatures for different types of bones. If the bones are a light golden brown and the meat is just barely browned, you have done it perfectly. If not, check them every 5 minutes until they're the desired color. The point of roasting is not to fully cook the ingredients but just give them a deeper flavor.

Where to Get Bones

Because of the recent renaissance of bone broth, it is near impossible to source any free bones these days. I have noticed that grocery stores are stocking more raw ingredients like chicken feet, beef bones, pork bones, and others. Check your local premium market for these ingredients in their butcher or frozen section. Or support local family-run farms who use responsible raising practices. Do you have a good local butcher in the area? I am sure they'd be happy to sell you their bones and feet for a fraction of what you would pay for lean cuts of meat. If you can't find anything locally, check online. There are a number of ranchers who team up to deliver bones direct to your doorstep. Remember, sourcing the best quality bones available is essential for receiving the health benefits of bone broth.

Core Ingredients

To make a truly delicious bone broth, it is important to use certain ingredients in every batch. Due to the intensity of the cooking process, the quality of all the ingredients must be extremely high. If the animals you are using were given steroids or other unnatural supplements or toxins during their life, you will absorb it directly through your bone broth. I will highlight some additional core ingredients in the following list, but it's important to remember to use meat along with bones in your recipes. If you can work directly with a butcher, ask for bones with meat and gristle attached. Feet are an excellent source of collagen and should be included in every bone broth recipe if possible. Chicken feet are fairly easy to source, but you may have to work harder to find a good source of beef and pork feet. (This is when making friends with your local butcher could prove beneficial!) Apple cider vinegar is vital to the overall quality of bone broth because it works to pull out the nutrients from the bones. It is best to pour the apple cider vinegar over the roasted meat and bones and allow it to sit for a few minutes prior to filling the pot with water. I use this technique in the recipes that follow but it bears mentioning here. If you source the following core ingredients from reputable and responsible suppliers, you will be very successful making bone broth:

- Chicken backs
- Chicken, beef, and pork feet
- Bones (femur, knuckle, back, ribs, etc.)
- Meat (shank, short ribs, etc.)
- Apple cider vinegar, raw and unfiltered
- Filtered water, fluoride free
- Vegetables

Essential Equipment

The process of cooking bone broth does not require fancy equipment. Aside from the chinois, you probably have all of the other equipment already on hand. Let's go over the essential equipment to make bone broth successfully.

ROASTING PAN: You want to make sure the pan you select has tall edges to catch any grease that collects at the bottom of the pan. I suggest lining the bottom with aluminum foil for easy cleanup.

KNIFE: You'll want a good sharp knife to chop vegetables and cut down any large chunks of meat into smaller pieces for more surface area.

POT: A stainless steel pot with a lid is a must for making your own bone broth. Due to the 24-hour cooking process, it's important to have a sturdy pot that you can trust. I typically choose one with a thick bottom for the most even cooking. In regard to size, ideally you would use a pot that holds at least 20 quarts, with a lid, for the best bone broth yield. A 6-quart pot would be the smallest useful size.

STRAINER: For the initial strain, you'll want to have a heavy-duty metal strainer with a sturdy handle.

CHINOIS: The chinois is a fine-mesh strainer, which gives you a more filtered bone broth. It will catch any debris not originally caught by the first strainer. You'll use the chinois for the second strain. You can also substitute it with cheesecloth if that's easier for you to source.

COMPOST BIN: Because you'll have plenty of food scraps, a good compost or food waste bin would be ideal. It's best for waste reduction and containment.

PATIENCE: Cooking bone broth is a process. Please be patient when cooking it for the first time.

Cooking Methods

One of my favorite parts about making my own bone broth is the variety of cooking methods. Some prefer to use a slow cooker or pressure cooker, while others like making it on the stovetop. Because bone broth is a traditional food, I believe the best way to make bone broth is with traditional methods. By simmering bone broth over low heat on the stovetop for a long time, you are able to get the most nutrients from the ingredients you use. This is a philosophy that will consistently yield a thick and gelatinous bone broth that's full of flavor. However, you can choose any method you prefer. If you're nervous about leaving bone broth unattended on the stovetop while you sleep or while you're at work, a slow cooker may work best. Alternatively, if you are making soup and require bone broth in a short amount of time, the pressure cooker may be your best option.

Cooking Method	Cooking Times	Best For
Stovetop	24 hours over low heat	All bone broth varieties
Slow Cooker	24 hours over low heat	Chicken and turkey
Pressure Cooker	2 hours under high pressure	Pork and beef

Evaluating Your Broth

The hard work is over. Your broth is cooked and cooled and now you're staring at its beauty. How do you know if you have made a proper nutrient-dense and flavorful bone broth? There are a few characteristics you should notice about your masterpiece.

JELL-O-LIKE CONSISTENCY: The most important characteristic of high-quality bone broth is the amount of gelatin present. When you shake the pot, the bone broth should be thick and difficult to move. This is the number one sign that you have cooked it correctly. If your bone broth does not gel, next time you should try one or all of these tips:

- Use less water. The ingredients should only be covered by 1 to 1½ inches of water when you begin the roasting process.
- Cook over a more consistent heat. Maybe your stove was set too low or too high. You're looking for a slight jiggle in the bubbles, not a roaring boil or, even worse, no bubbles at all.

SMELL: Bone broth should taste and smell good. I have heard some people complain about the smell of their bone broth while it's cooking. This is a direct result of sourcing ingredients that were conventionally raised. If the smell of your broth doesn't make your mouth water, then you should consider sourcing responsibly raised and organic ingredients next time.

CLARITY: This is a tricky one. How long you roast your meat and bones and whether they become charred will directly affect the color of the bone broth. If it is extremely dark, consider roasting the bones and meat at a lower temperature and for slightly less time. If your bone broth is extremely light in color, consider roasting the bones and meat at a higher temperature for slightly more time.

FLAVOR: Bone broth should be flavorful without the addition of salt. If it tastes "chalky," consider using fewer bones and more meat. If the broth lacks depth of flavor, consider adding more vegetables and herbs. The clarity will certainly play a role in flavor. If the clarity is too light, your bone broth will have a lighter flavor and vice versa.

Storing and Thawing Your Broth

The best way to store bone broth is in an airtight container. If you can consume it within a week, it's best to keep it all in the refrigerator. Otherwise, you can store it in the freezer for up to six months. If you're doing the diet plan, you shouldn't have any issue consuming all of the broth within a week. But, if you're at the tail end of it and want to save some for later, feel free to freeze it until you're ready to use it. The best way to thaw frozen bone broth is overnight in the refrigerator. But, if you're in a pinch, you can put the entire airtight container into a bowl of warm water to thaw.

Bone Broth FAQs

In the world of bone broth, there are questions someone new to bone broth might have.

Is there a difference between stock and broth?
To the purist, yes, there is a difference between stock and broth. Technically, stock is defined as bones and water simmered over low heat for a long time. Broth is technically meat and vegetables simmered over low heat for a long time. Bone broth is the best of both worlds since it combines bones, meat, vegetables, and herbs in water and is simmered for a long time.

Can I reuse bones to make more bone broth?
Some sources say you can reuse bones to make more broth. However, I suggest using fresh bones for each batch. As you slowly simmer your bone broth for an extended period of time, the nutrients from those bones are pulled out and left in the liquid. If you do it right, you shouldn't have many minerals or nutrients left in the bones after you're done using them in your first batch.

Can I feed my leftover meat or bones to my dog or cat?
Do not feed them any bones! Once bones are cooked, they can easily break apart and hurt your pet's digestive system. You can feed them some of the leftover meat, but you have to be careful. If you used any garlic or onions to make the broth, do not share any of that meat. I would only feed your pet a large chunk of meat if it's free of all other ingredients. Rinsing it under water could be helpful. Please use your best judgement here.

Can I feed my broth to my dog or cat?
Bone broth is great for your pet! It helps their gut health, which is incredibly sensitive. It also works well to keep their joints lubricated, helping them stay active for longer. Just make sure you do not use any onions or garlic in the bone broth, as they can't eat those vegetables.

Can I microwave my bone broth?
I highly recommend you warm your bone broth up on the stovetop. It only takes a few minutes and you can completely control the temperature and remove it as soon as it begins to bubble. Because gelatin is fragile, it's ideal to slowly warm it versus zapping it with the microwave.

Can I take bone broth on the go?
Absolutely! The best way to do this is to warm up bone broth in a saucepan until it just begins to boil. Then, transfer it to a thermal mug with a tight seal. There are some excellent ones on the market that keep bone broth hot for up to eight hours. Bone broth is the perfect afternoon snack!

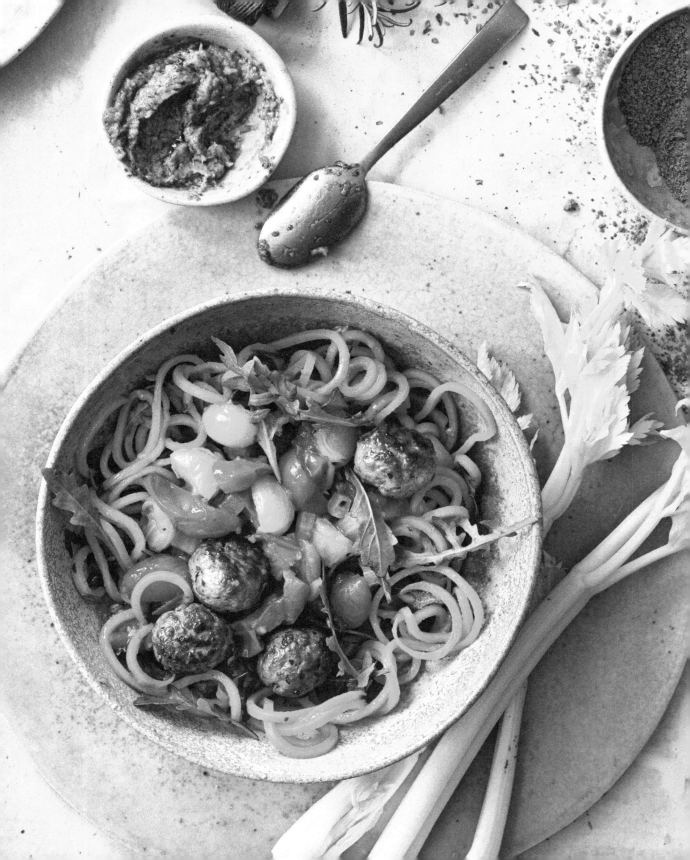

CHAPTER THREE

kick-starting the bone broth diet

The beauty of the 7-day bone broth diet is that you can start it whenever you want to without any additional commitment. The best part of the diet is that it's unlike any diet you have undertaken before. That's because the goal of it is to flood your system with the most nutrient-dense foods available, so you should not feel hungry while on the diet! The most important thing you can do to prepare is ensure you have plenty of whole foods available so you are not tempted to "cheat" by eating processed foods and sugars.

Preparing for the Diet

Most have achieved success on this diet with support from their family and friends. I recommend finding a friend or family member who would be interested in doing the diet with you. You can make it fun by preparing a few meals together and swapping. For instance, one of you can make chicken bone broth and the other can make beef bone broth. Then, you can share and have some variety throughout the cleanse. You can also each make a soup recipe and share half of it with the other person to add a little variety to the week. Plus, you can keep each other honest during the week and gab about the time you were tempted to eat cake but didn't.

Pick a Day to Start

I highly recommend you start the cleanse on a Sunday. You'll then have time to prepare all of the ingredients for the week ahead. If you can dedicate Saturday to grocery shopping and meal prep, you most certainly can begin on Sunday and be ready for the week.

Prepare Your Mind and Body

If you want to succeed at anything (including this diet), you have to be prepared. Cutting out processed food and sugar isn't easy for anyone. If you're not mentally and physically ready to go a full week nourishing your body with real food, then you will not be successful. If you're someone who needs a rigid schedule for eating or if you're habitually tied to certain foods not included on the diet, then you should begin weaning yourself off those foods the week prior to the cleanse. For example, I love eating Greek yogurt in the morning. But, because it's dairy and may contain sugar, it is not allowed on this plan. As a result, a few days prior to the cleanse, I eat eggs and bone broth instead. In order to help you transition off dairy I suggest choosing low or nonfat dairy equivalents (soy, rice, or almond milk, for example) with little to no added sugar.

If you regularly consume caffeine and alcohol, try eliminating it a week prior to the diet. You may experience some withdrawal symptoms, and it would help to start the diet without these toxins for the best results. If you find that you need to gently wean off alcohol and sugar, you may want to wait an additional week before starting the diet.

Diet FAQs

It is natural for you to have a few questions and concerns both before starting the diet and while you are in the middle of it. It is a new thing so don't be worried. Let's go over some commonly asked questions about this bone broth diet.

How will I feel on the first day?
You should feel great on the first day! You will notice yourself reaching for some of the foods you're used to, such as creamer or wine. But stand strong. After all, it's only a week, and in order to experience the best results, you should avoid all processed foods and sugars. You'll be shocked at how filling bone broth is! By replacing your morning coffee or evening wine with bone broth, you'll enjoy life in a whole new way. But you must strictly follow the rules for the 7-day bone broth diet to work effectively.

Should I only eat and use organic fruits and vegetables?
Organic ingredients are generally preferred and should be used whenever possible. Part of the goal of this diet is to maximize our intake of vitamins and nutrients, and organic foods provide more healthy benefits than nonorganic options. Even though the recipes do not specifically state you should use organic ingredients, try to purchase organic fruits, vegetables, and herbs as often as your budget allows.

Can I go to work while I am on this diet?
Absolutely! You should go about your normal activities. But listen to your body. If you're experiencing heavy withdrawal symptoms, or incredibly low energy, be sure to get some rest. Maybe your body has needed it and you have been ignoring the signs all along. Because bone broth is portable, I highly recommend bringing a portable insulated container full of already warmed bone broth to work with you. This will help you avoid cravings and keep you full.

Can I exercise during the diet?
If you were exercising prior to the 7-day bone broth cleanse and you're feeling up to it, go for it. If, like some, you experience an immense energy surge, you should absolutely burn it off with exercise. If you didn't exercise regularly prior to the 7-day bone broth cleanse and you're feeling up to it, please do. A light to moderate workout is excellent for keeping your energy levels up and your blood moving. You know your body best, so please use your best judgement.

Can I extend the diet?

If you're loving the 7-day bone broth diet and want to continue it for another week, you most certainly should. The bone broth diet is designed to lead to lifestyle changes rather than be just a momentary diet. It's also great to completely remove all processed foods and sugars from your diet in the long term to experience life in a healthier way.

Can I shorten the diet?

There will be some who prefer to only do the cleanse for 2 or 3 days. If you decide to do that, I recommend drinking more bone broth for the duration of your detox so you flood your system with gut-healing broth. If you want to cut it early because it just isn't working for you, then stop when you need and come back to it when you're mentally prepared.

The 7-Day Bone Broth Menu

It is important to note that this is merely an example of what you could be eating throughout the week. It's important to listen to your body and eat when you're hungry. This isn't a "one size fits all" diet, but merely a guideline of how you could structure your meals throughout the day. This menu ensures that you're getting 40 ounces of bone broth per day. It's also important for your body to fast after dinner until breakfast. If you are feeling hungry during this time, drink some hot tea.

While this sample menu plan does not include water, it is important to drink water throughout the day. Water is the best detoxifier there is and costs you zero calories, not that you should be counting. The recommended intake of water per day is half your body weight in ounces. For instance, if you weigh 100 pounds, you should drink 50 ounces of water per day.

Sample Menu Plan

	Breakfast (8 a.m.)	Snack (10 a.m.)	Lunch (12 p.m.)	Snack (3 p.m.)	Dinner (6 p.m.)
DAY 1	20 ounces **High-Performance Bone Broth** (page 44)	¼ cup nuts	20 ounces **High-Performance Bone Broth**	1 apple or banana	**Maple Bacon Lentil Soup with Kale** (page 69)
DAY 2	20 ounces **High-Performance Bone Broth**	¼ cup nuts	**Maple Bacon Lentil Soup with Kale**	1 apple or banana	20 ounces **Avocado Bone Broth Smoothie** (page 49)
DAY 3	20 ounces **Avocado Bone Broth Smoothie**	¼ cup nuts	20 ounces **Faux Eggnog** (page 45)	1 apple or banana	**Smothered Cremini Mushrooms with Homestyle Brat Sausage** (page 119)
DAY 4	20 ounces **Avocado Bone Broth Smoothie**	10 ounces bone broth of choice	**Smothered Cremini Mushrooms with Homestyle Brat Sausage**	Small handful of pecans or walnuts	**Thai Carrot Soup** (page 76)
DAY 5	20 ounces **High-Performance Bone Broth**	1 apple or banana	**Thai Carrot Soup**	Small handful of pecans or walnuts	20 ounces **Faux Eggnog**
DAY 6	20 ounces **Avocado Bone Broth Smoothie**	¼ cup nuts	**Thai Carrot Soup**	10 ounces bone broth of choice	**Spicy Pineapple Pork Stir-Fry** (page 129)
DAY 7	20 ounces **High-Performance Bone Broth**	1 apple or banana	**Spicy Pineapple Pork Stir-Fry**	10 ounces bone broth of choice	**Thai Carrot Soup**

Shopping List

BROTH
- Bone broth of your choice, 37.5 cups

MEATS
- Bacon, 5 slices (no nitrites, nitrates, or sugar)
- Bratwurst, 4 (no nitrites, nitrates, or sugar)
- Pork chops, 4 pounds (pastured boneless)

FRUITS & VEGETABLES
- Apples or bananas, 5
- Avocados, 2
- Bell peppers, 2
- Broccoli florets, 1 cup
- Butternut squash (to make 1 cup zoodles)
- Carrots, 3 pounds
- Cauliflower, 1 head
- Celery, 1 stalk
- Cilantro, 1 bunch
- Cremini mushrooms, 1 cup
- Garlic, 1 head
- Lacinato kale, 1 bunch
- Lentils, 1 cup dried
- Onions, 4
- Serrano pepper, 1 (optional)

HERBS, NUTS, AND SPICES
- Black pepper
- Coriander
- Ginger
- Nutmeg
- Nuts, 1 cup (I prefer walnuts or pecans)
- Salt
- Thyme

CANNED AND PANTRY ITEMS
- Coconut aminos
- Coconut cream, 1 cup (the stiff portion on top of the coconut milk)
- Coconut milk, full-fat, 1 (13.5-ounce) can
- Coconut oil
- Fish sauce
- Ghee
- Maple syrup
- Pineapple chunks, 1 (14-ounce) can
- Pumpkin purée, ½ cup
- Red curry paste

Making Bone Broth Part of Your Life

At this point, you have completed the 7-day bone broth diet and it was a huge success! Incorporating bone broth into your diet from here on out does not need to be a big production, nor does it mean consuming as much as 40 ounces a day. Daily consumption is essential in order to experience the benefits you are looking for. Here are some ideas on how best to utilize bone broth in your daily routines.

A Glass a Day

It is recommended to consume 8 to 10 ounces of bone broth one to two times per day as regular maintenance. If you're like me, you may choose to have it midmorning. I love a warm mug of bone broth to hold me over until lunch. It fills my belly and keeps me focused. Consuming it at night is also great because the amino acids found in bone broth can help you sleep. It's high in protein too, which will help keep you full throughout the night. It's also great in the morning for those who don't require a large breakfast. If you incorporate it into a smoothie, it can keep you full until lunch. But no matter what time of day, as long as you're drinking bone broth daily, you'll benefit.

Bone Broth on the Go

My favorite way to enjoy bone broth is on the go. It's an excellent snack that leaves me satisfied without feeling the need to grab something that will make me feel ill, like donuts, chips, or lattes. By warming your bone broth up before you leave and transporting it in an insulated container, you'll be set, whatever the destination.

Restarting the 7-Day Diet

Ready to do the 7-day bone broth diet again? Maybe you just got back from vacation or are in a sugar haze after the holidays and need to reboot, or you had such a great experience your first time that you are ready to start it all over again. The best part about the 7-day diet is that you can start whenever you're ready. It's all about preparing ingredients ahead of time so access to nutrient-dense foods and bone broth is readily available. We have already done the hard work: please consult the Shopping List (page 24) for your trip to the grocery store. Feel free to swap out bone broth recipes for other recipes that you enjoy in part 2. This diet is not about restricting what you can eat and how much you can eat; it's about providing many options. You will never be hungry, because you can eat as much as you need.

Part Two

The Recipes

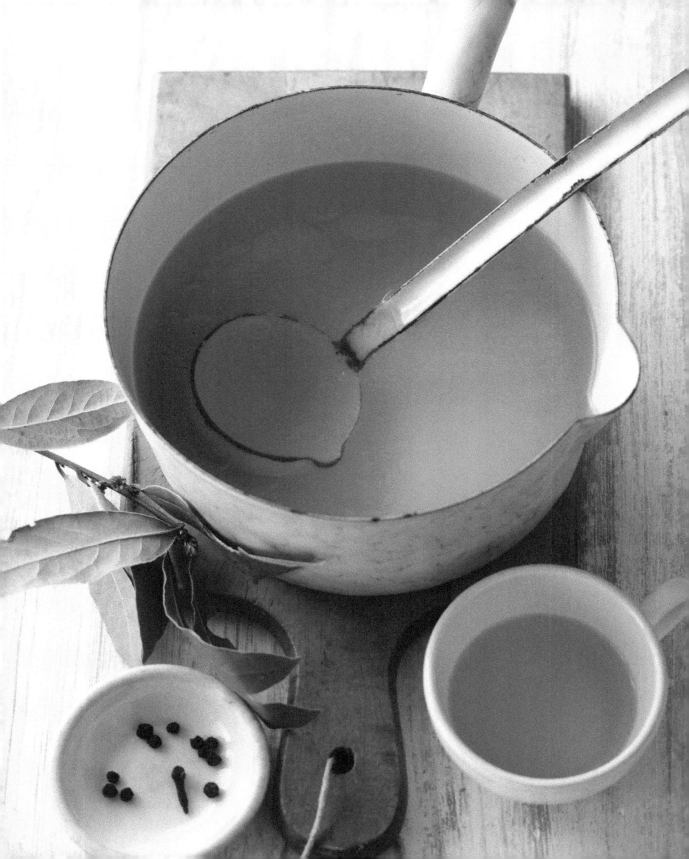

basic broths

(left) CHICKEN BONE BROTH, PAGE 30

chicken bone broth

DAIRY FREE · GLUTEN FREE · PALEO

MAKES ABOUT 10 CUPS **Known for its ability to cure even the slightest sniffle, chicken bone broth is a traditional kitchen staple all over the world. I personally love cooking dishes that contain chicken bone broth because of its subtle flavor. It is the best base for chicken noodle soup and an easy replacement for vegetable broth if you're seeking the benefits of gelatin. This recipe is a classic.**

PREP TIME: 30 minutes
STOVETOP: 18 to 24 hours
SLOW COOKER: 18 to 24 hours
PRESSURE COOKER: 2 hours

4 pounds pastured chicken feet
4 pounds pastured chicken backs
1 leek, trimmed
2 carrots
1 celery stalk
1 tablespoon apple cider vinegar
1 garlic clove
1 bunch thyme
1 tablespoon peppercorns
10 parsley sprigs
5 bay leaves
Filtered water

1. Preheat the oven to 425°F.

2. Line two roasting pans with aluminum foil and then top the foil with parchment paper. Divide the chicken feet and chicken backs between the two pans. Roast for 25 minutes, or until just slightly browned. It is better to undercook than overcook them.

3. While the chicken is roasting, chop the leek, carrots, and celery. Place the vegetables in the selected cooking pan and top with the roasted chicken.

4. Pour the apple cider vinegar on top and let sit for 5 minutes. Add the garlic, thyme, peppercorns, parsley, and bay leaves. Add just enough water to cover all the ingredients by only an inch.

5. Continue based on chosen cooking method.

STOVETOP

In a large pot over medium-high heat, heat the broth until bubbles begin to form, then lower the heat to its lowest setting. Cover the pot with a lid. Gently simmer for a minimum of 18 hours and a maximum of 24 hours. Ideally, your bone broth will cook between 190°F and 200°F. If necessary, only partially cover the broth while it simmers to avoid boiling and evaporation.

SLOW COOKER

Set to its lowest setting. Gently simmer, covered, for a minimum of 18 hours and a maximum of 24 hours. Ideally, your bone broth will cook between 190°F and 200°F.

PRESSURE COOKER

Manually set to 2 hours on high pressure. Vent and allow to normalize prior to removing the lid. After the broth has cooked, use a slotted spoon, tongs, or mesh strainer to remove all the ingredients from the liquid. After any large pieces of food are removed, pour the remaining liquid through a chinois and into a large container where it can be cooled. After 24 hours in the refrigerator, skim off the top layer of fat. The bone broth should jiggle with tons of gelatin and yummy flavor.

PREP TIP: It is important to cool your bone broth down prior to placing it in the refrigerator. I have found that an ice bath works really well. Pour a few inches of ice and water into the bottom of the sink. Place the sealed container in the sink, making sure the water is below the lip of the container. Drain the water and add fresh ice as necessary to keep the water ice cold. Once the bone broth has cooled to 75°F, you can place it in the refrigerator.

TIP: Why apple cider vinegar? Apple cider vinegar helps soften the bones and draw out the nutrients so you can consume them in the broth. The goal of making bone broth is to extract as many minerals and nutrients from the ingredients so you can reap the benefits. I enjoy using Bragg's Raw apple cider vinegar for its flavor, and because it's unfiltered and unpasteurized.

PER SERVING (1 CUP): CALORIES: 69; CARBS: 8G; SUGAR: 1G; FIBER: 1G; FAT: 2G; SATURATED FAT: 1G; PROTEIN: 5G; SODIUM: 10MG

beef bone broth

DAIRY FREE • GLUTEN FREE • PALEO

MAKES ABOUT 10 CUPS This recipe will yield a broth that is savory and satisfying. With the addition of tomatoes, this beef bone broth has a depth of flavor that is much richer than chicken. It's amazing sipped out of a mug or added to a hearty stew. Slightly higher in protein, this is one of my favorites. You will want this bone broth readily available at all times!

PREP TIME: 30 minutes

STOVETOP: 24 to 36 hours

SLOW COOKER: 24 to 36 hours

PRESSURE COOKER: 2 hours

3 pounds mixed grassfed beef bones (preferably a mix of long, knuckle, and neck)

1 pound grassfed beef brisket

2 pounds grassfed beef feet

1 onion

2 carrots

1 celery stalk

1 tablespoon apple cider vinegar

2 garlic cloves

1 bunch thyme

10 parsley sprigs

1 can whole peeled tomatoes

Filtered water

1. Preheat the oven to 425°F.

2. Line two roasting pans with aluminum foil and then top the foil with parchment paper. Divide the beef bones, brisket, and feet between the two pans. Roast for 20 minutes, or until just slightly browned. It is better to undercook than overcook them.

3. While the beef is roasting, chop the onion, carrots, and celery. Place the vegetables in the selected cooking pan with the roasted beef.

4. Pour the apple cider vinegar on top and let sit for 5 minutes. Add the garlic, thyme, parsley, and tomatoes. Add just enough water to cover all the ingredients by only an inch.

5. Continue based on chosen cooking method.

STOVETOP

In a large pot over medium-high heat, heat the broth until bubbles begin to form, then lower the heat to its lowest setting. Cover the pot with a lid. Gently simmer for a minimum of 24 hours and a maximum of 36 hours. Ideally, your bone broth will cook between 190°F and 200°F. If necessary, only partially cover the broth while it simmers to avoid boiling and evaporation.

SLOW COOKER

Set to its lowest setting. Gently simmer, covered, for a minimum of 24 hours and a maximum of 36 hours. Ideally, your bone broth will cook between 190°F and 200°F.

PRESSURE COOKER

1. Manually set to 2 hours on high pressure. Vent and allow to normalize prior to removing the lid.

2. After the broth has cooked, use a slotted spoon, tongs, or mesh strainer to remove all the ingredients from the liquid. After large pieces of food are removed, pour the remaining liquid through a chinois and into a large container where it can be cooled. After 24 hours in the refrigerator, skim off the top layer of fat. The bone broth should jiggle with tons of gelatin and yummy flavor.

PREP TIP: It is important to cool your bone broth down prior to placing it in the refrigerator. I have found that an ice bath works really well. Pour a few inches of ice and water into the bottom of the sink. Place the sealed container in the sink, making sure the water is below the lip of the container. Drain the water and add fresh ice as necessary to keep the water ice cold. Once the bone broth has cooled to 75°F, you can place it in the refrigerator.

ADD IN: Try rubbing the beef bones with tomato paste before cooking for added flavor.

PER SERVING (1 CUP): CALORIES: 80; CARBS: 4G; SUGAR: 2G; FIBER: 1G; FAT: 4G; SATURATED FAT: 1G; PROTEIN: 7G; SODIUM: 224MG

spicy pork bone broth

DAIRY FREE · GLUTEN FREE · PALEO

MAKES ABOUT 10 CUPS Add a little spice to tantalize your taste buds with this delicious recipe! This broth is the perfect addition to any recipe you'd like to add a little extra heat to. The original version of this uses habanero peppers, but feel free to substitute an extra jalapeño if the spice is too much to handle. I love using this bone broth as a marinade or to baste a roasted pork shoulder.

PREP TIME: 30 minutes
STOVETOP: 24 to 36 hours
SLOW COOKER: 24 to 36 hours
PRESSURE COOKER: 2 hours

3 pounds mixed pastured pork bones

2 pounds pastured pork shoulder

2 pounds pastured pig feet

2 onions

3 carrots

1 jalapeño pepper

1 poblano pepper

1 habanero (or substitute another jalapeño)

1 tablespoon apple cider vinegar

2 garlic cloves

10 parsley sprigs

1 can whole peeled tomatoes

Filtered water

1. Preheat the oven to 425°F.

2. Line two roasting pans with aluminum foil and then top the foil with parchment paper. Divide the pig bones, shoulder, and feet between the two pans. Roast for 25 minutes, or until just slightly browned. It is better to undercook than overcook them.

3. While the pork roasting, chop the onions, carrots, and peppers. Place the vegetables into the selected cooking pan, and top with the roasted pork.

4. Pour the apple cider vinegar on top and let sit for 5 minutes. Add the garlic, parsley, and tomatoes. Add just enough water to cover all the ingredients by only an inch.

5. Continue based on chosen cooking method.

STOVETOP

In a large pot over medium-high heat, heat the broth until bubbles begin to form, then lower heat to its lowest setting. Cover the pot with a lid. Gently simmer for a minimum of 24 hours and a maximum of 36 hours. Ideally, your bone broth will cook between 190°F and 200°F. If necessary, only partially cover the broth while it simmers to avoid boiling and evaporation.

SLOW COOKER

Set to its lowest setting. Gently simmer, covered, for a minimum of 24 hours and a maximum of 36 hours. Ideally, your bone broth will cook between 190°F and 200°F.

PRESSURE COOKER

1. Manually set to 2 hours on high pressure. Vent and allow to normalize prior to removing the lid.

2. After the broth has cooked, use a slotted spoon, tongs, or mesh strainer to remove all the ingredients from the liquid. After large pieces of food are removed, pour the remaining liquid through a chinois and into a large container where it can be cooled. After 24 hours in the refrigerator, skim off the top layer of fat. The bone broth should jiggle with tons of gelatin and yummy flavor.

PREP TIP: It is important to cool your bone broth down prior to placing it in the refrigerator. I have found that an ice bath works really well. Pour a few inches of ice and water into the bottom of the sink. Place the sealed container in the sink, making sure the water is below the lip of the container. Drain the water and add fresh ice as necessary to keep the water ice cold. Once the bone broth has cooled to 75°F, you can place it in the refrigerator.

TIP: Parsley is more than just a garnish. It is known for its vitamin K content, which has been linked to the promotion of bone growth and reduction of neuronal damage in the brain. Parsley has three times more vitamin C and A than an orange. It also contains iron, copper, and manganese and is known to detoxify the body. It's perfect for our 7-day diet.

PER SERVING (1 CUP): CALORIES: 72; CARBS: 3G; SUGAR: 2G; FIBER: 1G; FAT: 3G; SATURATED FAT: 1G; PROTEIN: 6G; SODIUM: 218MG

bison bone broth

DAIRY FREE · GLUTEN FREE · PALEO

MAKES ABOUT 10 CUPS I love this recipe because it's full of umami. With the addition of chicken feet to balance out the richness of the bison meat, its flavor is sure to impress. It's great for those of you who have allergies to beef but still love the richness that red meat offers. It's not gamey but has depth of flavor that you will love!

PREP TIME: 30 minutes
STOVETOP: 24 to 36 hours
SLOW COOKER: 24 to 36 hours
PRESSURE COOKER: 2 hours 15 minutes

4 pounds mixed grassfed bison bones (preferably a mix of long, knuckle, and neck)
1 pound grassfed bison brisket
2 pounds pastured chicken feet
1 onion
2 carrots
1 celery stalk
1 tablespoon apple cider vinegar
3 garlic cloves, chopped
½ bunch thyme
10 parsley sprigs
1 can whole peeled tomatoes
Filtered water

1. Preheat the oven to 425°F.

2. Line two roasting pans with aluminum foil and then top the foil with parchment paper. Divide the bison bones, bison brisket, and chicken feet between the two pans. Roast for 25 minutes, or until just slightly browned. It is better to undercook than overcook them.

3. While the bison and chicken are roasting, chop the onion, carrots, and celery. Place the vegetables in the selected cooking pan, and top with the roasted bison and chicken.

4. Pour the apple cider vinegar on top and let sit for 5 minutes. Add the garlic, thyme, parsley, and tomatoes. Add just enough water to cover all the ingredients by only an inch.

5. Continue based on chosen cooking method.

STOVETOP

In a large pot over medium-high heat, heat the broth until bubbles begin to form, then lower the heat to its lowest setting. Cover the pot with a lid. Gently simmer for a minimum of 24 hours and a maximum of 36 hours. Ideally, your bone broth will cook between 190°F and 200°F. If necessary, only partially cover the broth while it simmers to avoid boiling and evaporation.

SLOW COOKER

Set to its lowest setting. Gently simmer, covered, for a minimum of 18 hours and a maximum of 24 hours. Ideally, your bone broth will cook between 190°F and 200°F.

PRESSURE COOKER

1. Manually set to 2 hours 15 minutes on high pressure. Vent and allow to normalize prior to removing the lid.

2. After the broth has cooked, use a slotted spoon, tongs, or mesh strainer to remove all the ingredients from the liquid. After large pieces of food are removed, pour the remaining liquid through a chinois and into a large container where it can be cooled. After 24 hours in the refrigerator, skim off the top layer of fat. The bone broth should jiggle with tons of gelatin and yummy flavor.

PREP TIP: It is important to cool your bone broth down prior to placing it in the refrigerator. I have found that an ice bath works really well. Pour a few inches of ice and water into the bottom of the sink. Place the sealed container into the sink, making sure the water is below the lip of the container. Drain the water and add fresh ice as necessary to keep the water ice cold. Once the bone broth has cooled to 75°F, you can place it in your refrigerator.

PER SERVING (1 CUP): CALORIES: 65; CARBS: 4G; SUGAR: 2G; FIBER: 1G; FAT: 1G; SATURATED FAT: 0G; PROTEIN: 10G; SODIUM: 213MG

turkey bone broth

DAIRY FREE · GLUTEN FREE · PALEO

MAKES ABOUT 10 CUPS Thanksgiving is my favorite holiday. It's full of food, friends, and family. There's just something about the holiday that makes the turkey seem to taste better that day. Turkey bone broth gives me that same feeling. It is buttery and light, yet full of flavor. I love sipping on turkey bone broth before bed for its calming effects. You're going to enjoy this recipe throughout the year!

PREP TIME: 30 minutes
STOVETOP: 18 to 24 hours
SLOW COOKER: 18 to 24 hours
PRESSURE COOKER: 2 hours

2 pounds pastured chicken feet
4 pounds pastured turkey backs
1 leek, trimmed
2 carrots
1 celery stalk
1 tablespoon apple cider vinegar
1 garlic clove
1 bunch rosemary
10 parsley sprigs
Filtered water

1. Preheat the oven to 400°F.

2. Line two roasting pans with aluminum foil and then top the foil with parchment paper. Divide the chicken feet and turkey backs between the two pans. Roast for 20 minutes, or until just slightly browned. It is better to undercook than overcook them.

3. While the chicken and turkey are roasting, chop the leek, carrots, and celery. Place the vegetables in the selected cooking pan, and top with the roasted chicken feet and turkey backs.

4. Pour the apple cider vinegar on top and let sit for 5 minutes. Add the garlic, rosemary, and parsley. Add just enough water to cover all the ingredients by only an inch.

5. Continue based on chosen cooking method.

STOVETOP

In a large pot over medium-high heat, heat the broth until bubbles begin to form, then lower the heat to its lowest setting. Cover with a lid. Gently simmer for a minimum of 18 hours and a maximum of 24 hours. Ideally, your bone broth will cook between 190°F and 200°F. If necessary, only partially cover the broth while it simmers to avoid boiling and evaporation.

SLOW COOKER

Set to its lowest setting. Gently simmer, covered, for a minimum of 18 hours and a maximum of 24 hours. Ideally, your bone broth will cook between 190°F and 200°F.

PRESSURE COOKER

1. Manually set to 2 hours on high pressure. Vent and allow to normalize prior to removing the lid.

2. After the broth has cooked, use a slotted spoon, tongs, or mesh strainer to remove all the ingredients from the liquid. After large pieces of food are removed, pour the remaining liquid through a chinois and into a large container where it can be cooled. After 24 hours in the refrigerator, skim off the top layer of fat. The bone broth should jiggle with tons of gelatin and yummy flavor.

PREP TIP: It is important to cool bone broth down prior to placing it in the refrigerator. I have found that an ice bath works really well. Pour a few inches of ice and water into the bottom of the sink. Place the sealed container in the sink, making sure the water is below the lip of the container. Drain the water and add fresh ice as necessary to keep the water ice cold. Once the bone broth has cooled to 75°F, you can place it in the refrigerator.

SWAP TIP: It can be hard sourcing a good supply of turkey feet, so I created this recipe with that in mind. Feel free to use turkey feet if you can find them. Poultry feet are important in every recipe for the amount of gelatin they contain.

PER SERVING (1 CUP): CALORIES: 62; CARBS: 3G; SUGAR: 1G; FIBER: 1G; FAT: 2G; SATURATED FAT: 1G; PROTEIN: 8G; SODIUM: 33MG

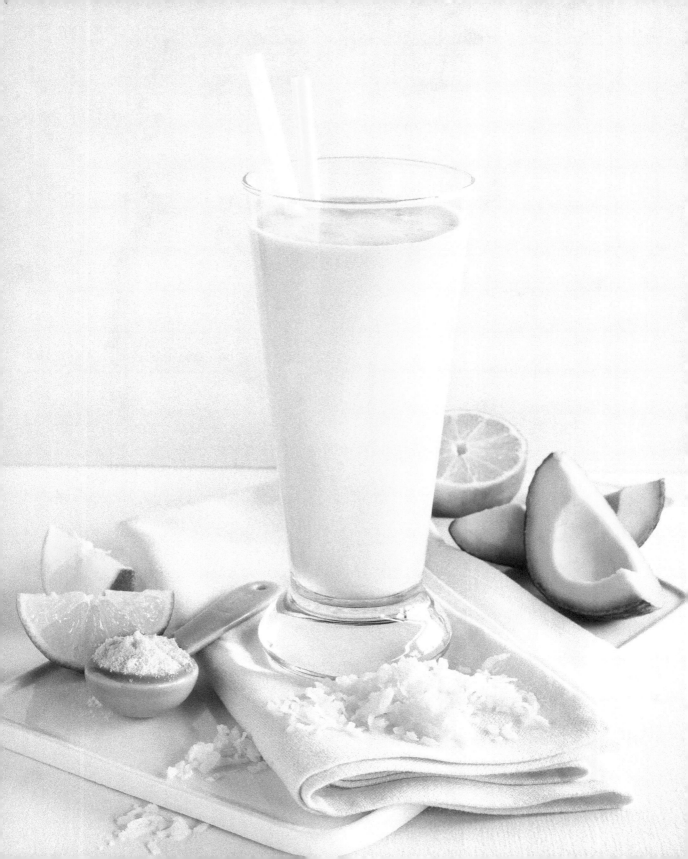

sipping drinks

(left) PUT THE LIME IN THE COCONUT, PAGE 52

broffee

DAIRY FREE • GLUTEN FREE • PALEO • QUICK & EASY

MAKES 1 SERVING I am going to be honest here. When I first heard of this concoction, I thought there was no way it could taste good. It was introduced to me by Dane, the director of customer experience at my company Osso Good. It's perfect to enjoy on the run in the morning because you can combine both your coffee and bone broth in one mug for an added energy kick. It works well with Chicken Bone Broth (page 30) or Turkey Bone Broth (page 38).

PREP TIME: 5 minutes

1 cup coffee, light to medium roast is best
1 cup bone broth, light flavor is best

Combine the coffee and broth in your favorite mug or your travel mug if you are on the go.

ADD IN: Add 1 tablespoon of coconut cream to make your Broffee creamier.

PER SERVING: CALORIES: 27; CARBS: 0G; SUGAR: 0G; FIBER: 1G; FAT: 1G; SATURATED FAT: 0G; PROTEIN: 6G; SODIUM: 300MG

pumpkin pie smoothie

DAIRY FREE • GLUTEN FREE • PALEO • QUICK & EASY

MAKES 1 SERVING If you love pumpkin pie, you're sure to love this recipe! It's loaded with those comforting fall flavors we wait all year to enjoy. The honey is listed as optional because while you're on the diet, it's important to consume honey in moderation. But honey is a perfectly natural way to sweeten this fall beverage.

PREP TIME: 5 minutes

10 ounces Chicken Bone Broth (page 30) or Beef Bone Broth (page 32)

1 teaspoon pumpkin pie spice (see Tip)

½ cup pumpkin purée

¼ cup coconut cream (the solid part in coconut milk, naturally sweet)

1 teaspoon raw, unfiltered honey (optional)

Add all the ingredients to your blender and purée.

PREP TIP: Many stores sell a version of pumpkin pie spice, but you can make your own to use not only in this recipe, but in others throughout the holiday season, too.

PUMPKIN PIE SPICE:
3 tablespoons ground cinnamon
2 teaspoons ground ginger
2 teaspoons ground nutmeg
1½ teaspoons ground allspice
1½ teaspoons ground cloves

Combine all the ingredients and mix. Keep stored in an airtight container in your spice cabinet.

PER SERVING: CALORIES: 223; CARBS: 16G; SUGAR: 10G; FIBER: 5G; FAT: 13G; SATURATED FAT: 11G; PROTEIN: 15G; SODIUM: 20MG

high-performance bone broth

GLUTEN FREE • PALEO • QUICK & EASY

MAKES 1 SERVING **This broth is one of my favorites. It's simple, yet filling. Best of all, it really gives you an energy kick! The fat in the ghee mixed with the bone broth keeps you full longer, too. This is perfect as a replacement for your morning coffee if you'd prefer to remove caffeine from your diet.**

PREP TIME: 5 minutes

10 ounces bone broth (my favorite variety to use in this recipe is Beef Bone Broth, page 32)

1 tablespoon ghee

Pinch sea salt

In a medium saucepan over medium heat, warm the broth until it just starts to bubble. Pour the warm broth into a large mug. Add the ghee and salt. Use a whisk or handheld frother to fully mix the ingredients. Serve and be prepared for an energy kick!

ADD IN: For an extra flavor kick, add 1 teaspoon of ground cinnamon.

PER SERVING: CALORIES: 185; CARBS: 0G; SUGAR: 0G; FIBER: 0G; FAT: 15G; SATURATED FAT: 9G; PROTEIN: 12G; SODIUM: 0MG

faux eggnog

MAKES 1 SERVING This is one of my favorite ways to enjoy bone broth over the holidays! It's not quite as thick as eggnog, but I consider this beverage to be "Christmas in a cup." It's best served immediately after frothing to enjoy the thick layer of foam on top. This beverage is full of anti-inflammatory ingredients. Plus, nutmeg is known for its ability to eliminate bad breath, so add in a little extra if you might end up under the mistletoe.

PREP TIME: 5 minutes

8 ounces bone broth

½ cup coconut cream

1 tablespoon coconut oil

1 tablespoon ghee

1 teaspoon ground nutmeg

Pinch sea salt

In a medium saucepan over medium heat, warm the broth until it just starts to bubble. Pour the warm broth into a large mug. Add the coconut cream, coconut oil, ghee, nutmeg, and salt. Use a whisk or handheld frother to fully mix, then serve.

PER SERVING: CALORIES: 547; CARBS: 3G; SUGAR: 1G; FIBER: 0G; FAT: 55G; SATURATED FAT: 43G; PROTEIN: 12G; SODIUM: 185MG

mango smoothie

DAIRY FREE • GLUTEN FREE • PALEO • QUICK & EASY

MAKES 1 SERVING This smoothie is perfect as a cool way to sip your bone broth in the summer. The custard-like texture of the mango increases the thickness of the smoothie. I like to double this recipe and freeze the second portion for a frozen treat midafternoon when the sunlight is at its most intense.

PREP TIME: 5 minutes

10 ounces Chicken Bone Broth (page 30)
½ large ripe mango, cut into chunks
Pinch sea salt

Add all the ingredients to your blender and purée.

PER SERVING: CALORIES: 123; CARBS: 18G; SUGAR: 14G; FIBER: 2G; FAT: 1G; SATURATED FAT: 0G; PROTEIN: 12G; SODIUM: 115MG

orange you beet

DAIRY FREE • GLUTEN FREE • PALEO • QUICK & EASY

MAKES 2 SERVINGS **The sweetness of the beet paired with the citrus of the orange is perfect in this bone broth smoothie. It is bright in flavor and the natural sugars in the beet will keep your heart pumping. This is great to drink right before a workout.**

PREP TIME: 5 minutes

10 ounces Chicken Bone Broth (page 30)

1 large beet, roasted

Juice of 1 large orange

Juice of ½ lemon

1 teaspoon honey

In a small saucepan over medium heat, warm the broth until it just starts to bubble. Put all the ingredients into a blender and pulse on high until the beet is well macerated. Enjoy!

PER SERVING: CALORIES: 56; CARBS: 7G; SUGAR: 5G; FIBER: 1G; FAT: 1G; SATURATED FAT: 0G; PROTEIN: 6G; SODIUM: 128MG

Bone Broth Add-Ins

In and of itself, bone broth is full of nutrients and flavor, but additional ingredients can give these an extra oomph in both departments—especially if you're drinking a cup (or more) of broth daily.

Turmeric

Turmeric, a bright yellow root that's commonly used in Indian cuisine, is one of the most effective natural reducers of inflammation. Add 2 to 4 2-inch-long, finger-size pieces of fresh turmeric to your pot along with the bones or stir a tablespoon or so of ground turmeric in to hot broth.

Ginger

Zingy ginger root aids digestion, soothes nausea, and helps reduce flatulence. Like turmeric, ginger also has anti-inflammatory properties. Add a chopped 3-inch piece of fresh ginger to your bone broth recipe along with the bones before simmering. Ground ginger can be stirred into hot broth just before serving.

Seaweed

Simmer a few strips of seaweed in your bone broth for extra umami, and you'll also get additional vitamins like A, B, C, E, and K, as well as important minerals like iodine, selenium, calcium, and iron. Add 2 or 3 pieces of kombu, kelp, or wakame seaweed to your pot along with the water and bones before bringing to a simmer.

Wild Mushrooms

Mushrooms impart earthy flavors, and their glucans also help boost the immune system and protect against viruses, bacteria, and possibly even cancer. Add dried or fresh mushrooms—shiitake, porcini, or others—to the pot along with the bones and water before simmering.

avocado bone broth smoothie

DAIRY FREE • GLUTEN FREE • PALEO • QUICK & EASY

MAKES 2 SERVINGS This recipe was created by my husband, Jazz, and it's absolutely delicious! He loves adding a splash of hot sauce to it for an added kick. The healthy fats in the avocado keep you full for hours and the cilantro tastes super fresh. I love drinking this smoothie on the road. This recipe will yield a double portion, so be sure to share it or save it for later. Serve with a squeeze of lime juice to add a tangy citrus flavor.

PREP TIME: 5 minutes

20 ounces bone broth

½ avocado

1 cup chopped fresh cilantro

½ teaspoon sea salt

In a medium saucepan over medium heat, warm the broth until it just starts to bubble. Add all the ingredients to a blender and blend until completely smooth. Enjoy!

PER SERVING: CALORIES: 140; CARBS: 6G; SUGAR: 1G; FIBER: 4G; FAT: 8G; SATURATED FAT: 1G; PROTEIN: 13G; SODIUM: 116MG

truffled pink smoothie

DAIRY FREE • GLUTEN FREE • PALEO • QUICK & EASY

MAKES 1 SERVING This recipe has earthy flavors that incorporate the healing power of mushrooms. Reishi mushrooms are one of the best sources of adaptogens on the planet, known for their ability to detox the body, calm the nerves, and boost immunity. I like to use pink Himalayan sea salt to round out the flavors.

PREP TIME: 5 minutes

10 ounces bone broth

1 tablespoon truffle oil

1 tablespoon reishi powder

½ teaspoon sea salt

In a medium saucepan over medium heat, warm the broth until it just starts to bubble. Whisk or froth all the remaining ingredients in to the warmed broth. Enjoy!

PER SERVING: CALORIES: 196; CARBS: 5G; SUGAR: 0G; FIBER: 5G; FAT: 15G; SATURATED FAT: 2G; PROTEIN: 12G; SODIUM: 1275MG

flu buster

DAIRY FREE • GLUTEN FREE • PALEO • QUICK & EASY

MAKES 1 SERVING **Drink this at the first sign you may be coming down with a cold or flu. It's bursting with immune-boosting ingredients that taste so good together. Chicken bone broth has been proven to enhance the immune system, and once you add in vitamin C from the lemon, honey's antiviral properties, and the minerals from sea salt, it's a delicious sickness-fighting combination!**

PREP TIME: 5 minutes

10 ounces Chicken Bone Broth (page 30)

1 tablespoon raw honey

1 tablespoon coconut oil

Juice of ½ lemon

Pinch sea salt

In a medium saucepan over medium heat, warm the broth until simmering. Whisk or froth all the remaining ingredients into the warmed broth. Enjoy!

PER SERVING: CALORIES: 256; CARBS: 19G; SUGAR: 18G; FIBER: 0G; FAT: 15G; SATURATED FAT: 13G; PROTEIN: 11G; SODIUM: 268MG

put the lime in the coconut

DAIRY FREE • GLUTEN FREE • PALEO • QUICK & EASY

MAKES 1 SERVING This recipe is perfect in the afternoon. It has a beautiful light taste with a punch of citrus to brighten your mood. The second sip is better than the first and it just keeps getting better.

PREP TIME: 5 minutes

8 ounces Chicken Bone Broth (page 30)

¼ cup coconut milk (liquid)

2 tablespoons coconut cream (the stiff part that separates in the coconut milk can)

Juice of ½ lime

Pinch Celtic sea salt

Cilantro leaves, chopped

In a small saucepan over medium heat, warm the broth until it just begins to bubble. Combine all the ingredients in a blender and blend until well mixed. Garnish with cilantro and serve immediately.

PER SERVING: CALORIES: 223; CARBS: 3G; SUGAR: 2G; FIBER: 0G; FAT: 18G; SATURATED FAT: 14G; PROTEIN: 10G; SODIUM: 268MG

spicy citrus

DAIRY FREE • GLUTEN FREE • PALEO • QUICK & EASY

MAKES 1 SERVING The ginger, pepper, and turmeric add a nice bite to this smooth citrus beverage. This recipe offers superfoods at their best. It's perfect for keeping the sniffles away and bright enough to wake you up in the morning.

PREP TIME: 5 minutes

20 ounces Turkey Bone Broth (page 38)

1 (2-inch) piece ginger, peeled

Juice of ½ lemon

½ teaspoon turmeric

½ teaspoon sea salt

½ teaspoon freshly ground black pepper

In a large saucepan over medium-low heat, bring all the ingredients to a simmer. Remove from the heat and pour into your favorite mug.

PER SERVING: CALORIES: 122; CARBS: 3G; SUGAR: 1G; FIBER: 0G; FAT: 2G; SATURATED FAT: 0G; PROTEIN: 23G; SODIUM: 1388MG

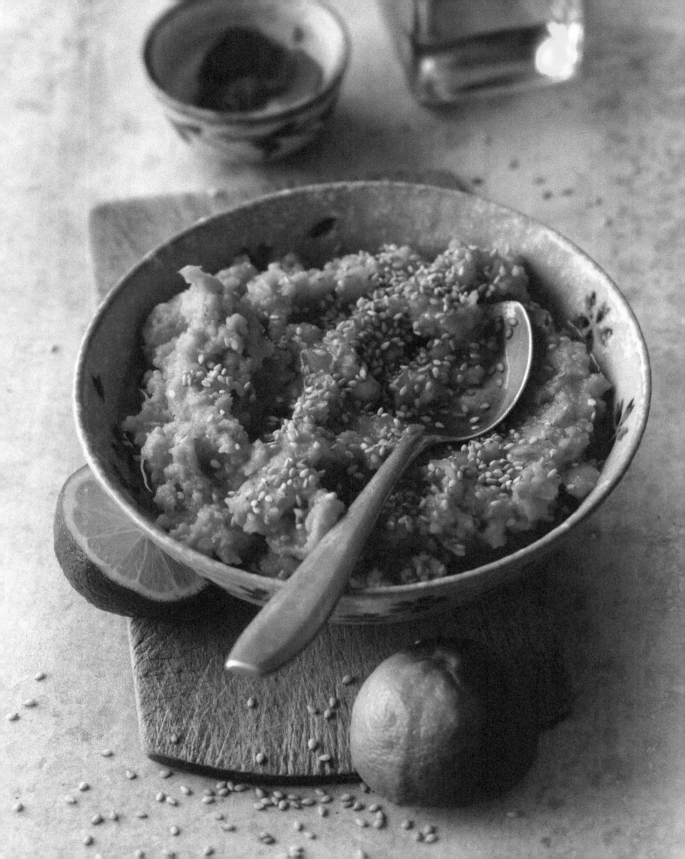

sides

(left) SWEET POTATO PURÉE, PAGE 62

guacamole

DAIRY FREE • GLUTEN FREE • PALEO • QUICK & EASY

MAKES 4 SERVINGS Every great party needs a great guacamole recipe. And by every party, I mean every meal. This is the creamiest guacamole I have ever tasted, hands down. Once you taste it, I am sure that you will agree.

PREP TIME: 10 minutes

3 ripe avocados

¾ cup bone broth

Juice of ½ lime

1 jalapeño pepper, finely chopped

1 small red onion, finely chopped

1 bunch cilantro, minced

Salt

Freshly ground black pepper

1. On a clean cutting board, cut the avocados in half, discard the pits, and scoop out the flesh.

2. In a medium bowl, mash the avocado and add the broth.

3. Add the lime juice, jalapeño, onion, and cilantro, and stir until combined. Season with salt and pepper before serving. Enjoy!

PER SERVING: CALORIES: 238; CARBS: 14G; SUGAR: 1G; FIBER: 10G; FAT: 20G; SATURATED FAT: 3G; PROTEIN: 5G; SODIUM: 28MG

lacinato kale

GLUTEN FREE • PALEO • QUICK & EASY

MAKES 4 SERVINGS **Kale is a magnificent vegetable. It is most nutritious when served cooked, so eat up! I love mixing it into mashed cauliflower or parsnips and topping everything with pomegranate seeds.**

PREP TIME: 5 minutes

COOK TIME: 5 minutes

20 ounces bone broth

**2 bunches lacinato kale, stemmed
    and chopped**

¼ teaspoon salt

¼ teaspoon freshly ground black pepper

¼ teaspoon garlic powder

1 teaspoon ghee

In a large saucepan over high heat, bring the broth to a boil. Add the kale. Cover and cook for 5 minutes. Add the salt, pepper, garlic powder, and ghee. Serve immediately.

PER SERVING: CALORIES: 74; CARBS: 7G; SUGAR: 0G; FIBER: 1G; FAT: 2G; SATURATED FAT: 1G; PROTEIN: 8G; SODIUM: 232MG

balsamic cherry reduction

GLUTEN FREE • PALEO • QUICK & EASY

MAKES 6 TO 8 SERVINGS **This balsamic cherry reduction is the perfect sauce to pour over any protein of your choice. I personally love it over Cajun Beef Brisket with Cherries (page 118) and Roasted Chicken Thighs (page 127). It is excellent with mashed sweet potatoes, too!**

PREP TIME: 5 minutes
COOK TIME: 30 minutes

2 cups frozen cherries
10 ounces Beef Bone Broth (page 32)
1 tablespoon balsamic vinegar
2 tablespoons ghee

1. In a medium saucepan over medium heat, combine all the ingredients. Bring to a gentle boil and reduce the heat to medium-low.

2. Cook, uncovered, until about half of the liquid has reduced, about 30 minutes.

3. Roughly mash the cherries and serve.

PER SERVING: CALORIES: 85; CARBS: 8G; SUGAR: 6G; FIBER: 1G; FAT: 5G; SATURATED FAT: 3G; PROTEIN: 3G; SODIUM: 1MG

cauliflower rice

DAIRY FREE • GLUTEN FREE • PALEO • QUICK & EASY

MAKES 6 TO 8 SERVINGS **When made the right way, this cauliflower rice is the perfect substitute for rice when cleansing. Cauliflower is an excellent source of vitamins C, K, and B$_6$. It's nourishing and delicious!**

PREP TIME: 5 minutes

COOK TIME: 10 minutes

20 ounces bone broth

1 cauliflower head, cut into florets

1. In a medium saucepan over high heat, bring the broth to a gentle boil and add the cauliflower florets. Cook, uncovered, for 10 minutes.

2. Strain, reserving the liquid, and use a potato masher to gently turn the cauliflower into rice.

BONE BROTH TIP: You can reserve the bone broth liquid to sip on right before bed. Or, save it to cook another veggie!

PER SERVING: CALORIES: 61; CARBS: 7G; SUGAR: 3G; FIBER: 4G; FAT: 0G; SATURATED FAT: 0G; PROTEIN: 9G; SODIUM: 43MG

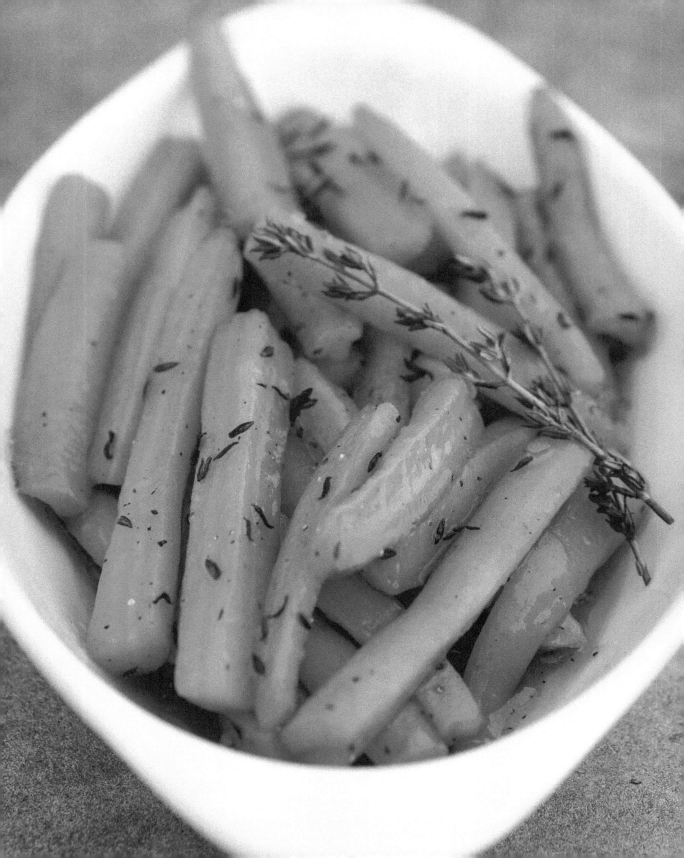

caramelized carrots

GLUTEN FREE • PALEO • QUICK & EASY

MAKES 8 SERVINGS **Caramelized carrots are mouthwatering and naturally sweet. I have been found eating them alone straight out of their dish, but they are a perfect complement to most dishes as a wonderful side. For a rich, herby flavor, serve with fresh thyme.**

PREP TIME: 5 minutes

COOK TIME: 15 minutes

½ cup bone broth

2 pounds carrots, quartered lengthwise

1 teaspoon sea salt, divided

¼ cup honey

¼ cup ghee

1 teaspoon orange peel

1. In a medium sauté pan over medium-low heat, combine the broth, carrots, and ½ teaspoon of salt. Simmer for about 12 minutes, or until the carrots are fork-tender.

2. In a medium saucepan over medium heat, heat the honey, ghee, orange peel, and the remaining ½ teaspoon of salt, stirring frequently.

3. Cook until the first bubbles form and then remove from the heat. Add the carrot and bone broth mixture to the saucepan and mix thoroughly. Enjoy!

PER SERVING: CALORIES: 149; CARBS: 20G; SUGAR: 14G; FIBER: 3G; FAT: 8G; SATURATED FAT: 4G; PROTEIN: 2G; SODIUM: 369MG

sweet potato purée

GLUTEN FREE • PALEO • QUICK & EASY

MAKES 10 SERVINGS This purée is a perfect addition to almost any meal. I love it on its own or topped with fresh pico de gallo. Sweet potato purée is not just for Thanksgiving anymore.

PREP TIME: 5 minutes

COOK TIME: 20 minutes

10 large sweet potatoes, peeled and chopped

6 ounces bone broth, warmed

2 tablespoons ghee

¼ cup coconut cream

½ teaspoon ground cinnamon

½ teaspoon salt

⅛ teaspoon ground nutmeg

Sesame seeds, for garnish (optional)

1. In a large pot over high heat, bring water to a boil and add the sweet potatoes. Cook for 15 to 20 minutes or until the potatoes are soft enough to puncture with a fork.

2. Drain the water from the pot and add the broth, ghee, coconut cream, cinnamon, salt, and nutmeg.

3. Mash with a potato masher. Serve garnished with sesame seeds, if desired. Enjoy!

SUBSTITUTION TIP: Use yams or purple sweet potatoes instead for a different color profile. You can also replace the ghee with 2 table-spoons of extra-virgin olive oil, replace the cinnamon and nutmeg with 1 teaspoon of paprika, and add 1 tablespoon of sesame seeds and 1 teaspoon of lime juice for a delicious spin on the classic recipe.

PER SERVING: CALORIES: 204; CARBS: 37G; SUGAR: 12G; FIBER: 6G; FAT: 4G; SATURATED FAT: 3G; PROTEIN: 3G; SODIUM: 189MG

parsnip purée

GLUTEN FREE • PALEO • QUICK & EASY

MAKES 4 SERVINGS Parsnips are sweet, like carrots, and make a great replacement for carbohydrate-rich potatoes. I personally love these on top of French Onion Soup (page 81).

PREP TIME: 5 minutes
COOK TIME: 15 minutes

20 ounces bone broth
1 pound parsnips, peeled and sliced
3 garlic cloves, smashed
2 teaspoons salt, divided
½ cup ghee
1 thyme sprig, stemmed
1 teaspoon onion powder with parsley
1 teaspoon freshly ground black pepper

1. In a large pot over high heat, combine the broth, parsnips, garlic, and 1 teaspoon of salt. Bring to a boil and then reduce the heat to medium-high so it becomes a gentle boil. Cook until tender, about 12 minutes.

2. Strain the parsnips and garlic, reserving the cooking liquid. Add the ghee, thyme, onion powder, the remaining 1 teaspoon of salt, and the pepper to the parsnips.

3. Begin mashing the parsnips with a potato masher and slowly add cooking liquid until you achieve a texture similar to whipped cream.

PER SERVING: CALORIES: 379; CARBS: 20G; SUGAR: 5G; FIBER: 4G; FAT: 30G; SATURATED FAT: 18G; PROTEIN: 8G; SODIUM: 1174MG

Bone Broth in Different Cultures

It's a hip menu item these days, but bone broth has figured in culinary and medicinal traditions around the world for eons, known both for its culinary value and its purported health benefits.

The Middle East

The Sephardic Jews of North Africa and other peoples of the Middle East have a documented history of making nourishing chicken soup for health. Back in the 12th century, the Jewish philosopher and physician Maimonides recommended chicken bone broth as both food and medicine in his book, *On the Cause of Symptoms*. When Jews migrated into Europe, they brought this dish with them, and eventually chicken soup became part of mainstream Jewish culture worldwide. But you don't have to be Jewish to offer up steaming bowls of chicken broth ladled over matzo balls or noodles anytime a family member gets a sniffle.

Eastern Europe

Variations of *borscht*, a beet soup with a bone broth base, can be found across Eastern Europe. In Ukraine's capital city, Kiev, it often includes bacon and beans. In the central city of Poltava, the broth is made from goose bones. Moscow borscht usually includes sausage, and in Lithuania, the soup is most often served cold.

Vietnam

When the French colonized Vietnam in the 18th century, they brought with them a love of beef. In the hands of Vietnamese cooks, beef bones became the foundation of what has become known as the national dish of Vietnam, *pho*—rice noodles in a rich broth made by simmering bones with ginger, star anise, and other spices.

Korea

Bone broth-based soups are common across Asia, where meals frequently include a clear broth as a palate cleanser and digestive aid. In Korea, *seolleongtang*—a hearty stew made from ox bones and beef brisket—is especially popular during the cold winter months.

France

Whether made from veal bones, beef bones, chicken or other poultry bones, bone broths are foundational ingredients in just about every traditional savory French sauce or soup.

The Caribbean

In the Caribbean, collagen-rich cow foot soup is a popular breakfast food, known for giving strength and as a cure-all for ailments.

bone broth hummus

DAIRY FREE • GLUTEN FREE • PALEO • QUICK & EASY

MAKES 12 SERVINGS **This bone broth hummus is an excellent snack. When I don't have time for a full meal or I am simply not hungry enough, having a few veggies on hand to dip into this hummus can be a lifesaver. It doesn't take much to fill you up and it keeps in the refrigerator for 7 to 10 days.**

PREP TIME: 10 minutes

1 cup presoaked chickpeas

6 tablespoons extra-virgin olive oil

Juice of 1 lemon

2 teaspoons sea salt

1 teaspoon ground cumin

2 tablespoons tahini

¼ cup bone broth

In a food processor, combine all the ingredients. Mix well until it has a smooth consistency. Serve with vegetables of your choice.

> TIP: My favorite vegetables to dip in hummus are carrots, jicama, cucumbers, and red peppers.

PER SERVING: CALORIES: 100; CARBS: 5G; SUGAR: 1G; FIBER: G1; FAT: 9G; SATURATED FAT: 1G; PROTEIN: 2G; SODIUM: 391MG

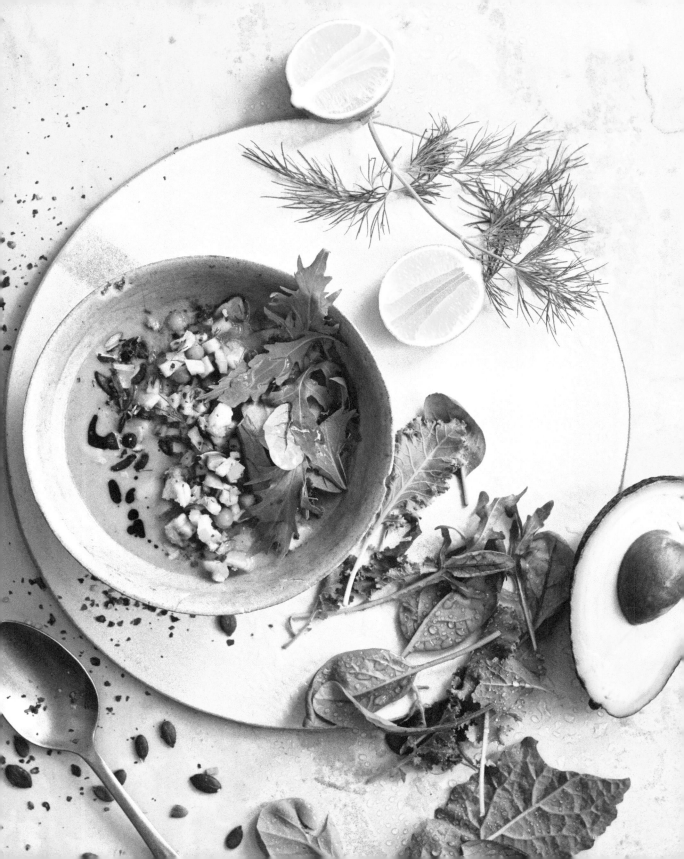

soups

(left) CREAMY PEA SOUP WITH AVOCADO AND APPLE SALSA, PAGE 82

sausage and kale soup
with roasted sweet potatoes

DAIRY FREE • GLUTEN FREE • PALEO

MAKES 4 SERVINGS I really enjoy this hearty soup during cooler weather or when I am ravenous on a summer morning. The best part about this soup is that it tastes even better the next day. The red pepper flakes are optional, but they add a good amount of heat to the dish if you like your soups spicy. You can use any bone broth you'd like for this recipe, but I prefer Spicy Pork Bone Broth (page 34) or Chicken Bone Broth (page 30).

PREP TIME: 10 minutes
COOK TIME: 40 minutes

2 tablespoons extra-virgin olive oil

2 sweet potatoes, cubed

4 teaspoons salt, divided

4 teaspoons freshly ground black pepper, divided

4 teaspoons garlic powder, divided

1 onion, chopped

2 garlic cloves, sliced

1 tablespoon coconut oil

1 pound ground pastured pork

40 ounces bone broth

4 cups kale, stemmed and chopped

½ teaspoon fresh thyme leaves

½ teaspoon red pepper flakes (optional)

1. Preheat the oven to 425°F.

2. In a roasting pan, drizzle the olive oil over the sweet potatoes. Season the potatoes with 2 teaspoons each of salt, pepper, and garlic powder. Roast for 10 to 20 minutes, flipping once. Set aside.

3. In a Dutch oven over medium heat, sauté the onion and garlic in the coconut oil for 5 minutes, stirring frequently.

4. Add the pork and the remaining 2 teaspoons of salt, breaking the pork into chunks with a large spoon. Cook for 5 minutes or until browned.

5. Add the broth, kale, sweet potatoes, thyme, red pepper flakes (if using), and the remaining 2 teaspoons each of pepper and garlic powder. Cook for 10 minutes more, and serve.

PER SERVING: CALORIES: 568; CARBS: 27G; SUGAR: 4G; FIBER: 4G; FAT: 36G; SATURATED FAT: 13G; PROTEIN: 34G; SODIUM: 2541MG

maple bacon lentil soup with kale

DAIRY FREE • GLUTEN FREE

MAKES 4 SERVINGS You are going to have a hard time believing that this soup is cleanse friendly! It is so good that every time I make it, I want to make it again the next day. The sweetness of the maple syrup paired with the earthy depth of the lentils is an unbeatable matchup. Full of flavor and nourishment, this will be a new weekly staple.

PREP TIME: 10 minutes, plus 8 hours to soak

COOK TIME: 40 minutes

1 cup dry lentils, soaked for at least
      8 hours

5 heritage bacon slices, cooked and chopped

1 onion, diced

1 garlic clove, sliced

2 carrots, diced

1 celery stalk, diced

1 teaspoon ground coriander

1 teaspoon salt

1 teaspoon freshly ground black pepper

20 ounces Beef Bone Broth (page 32)

½ cup pumpkin purée

1 tablespoon maple syrup

2 cups lacinato kale, stemmed and chopped

1. Drain the lentils and set aside.

2. In a Dutch oven over medium heat, place the bacon in a single layer on the bottom and cook for 1 to 2 minutes. Flip once so both sides are lightly browned. Remove and set aside.

3. In the bacon grease, cook the onion and garlic for 3 minutes, stirring frequently.

4. Add the carrots, celery, coriander, salt, and pepper. Cook for 3 minutes.

5. Add the broth, lentils, pumpkin purée, maple syrup, chopped bacon, and kale. Bring to a gentle boil and then reduce the heat to low. Simmer for 30 minutes, then serve.

PREP TIP: Soak your lentils for 8 hours. If you buy dried lentils and soak them in twice the amount of water with a pinch of salt, you will not be disappointed. They stay firm through the cooking process, versus canned lentils, which can sometimes turn to mush after cooking.

PER SERVING: CALORIES: 227; CARBS: 36G; SUGAR: 9G; FIBER: 15G; FAT: 5G; SATURATED FAT: 0G; PROTEIN: 21G; SODIUM: 803MG

thai coconut soup (tom kha)

DAIRY FREE • PALEO

MAKES 4 SERVINGS The infusion of ginger, garlic, and lemongrass in this soup adds subtle flavor, naturally. It's perfect year-round for a nourishing meal. I personally love finishing off a busy day with a bowl of this wonderful soup.

PREP TIME: 5 minutes

COOK TIME: 35 minutes

2 lemongrass stalks

1 ¼-inch piece fresh ginger, peeled

1 garlic clove

10 kaffir lime leaves

40 ounces Chicken Bone Broth (page 30)

2 pounds pastured chicken, cut into 1-inch pieces

1 (13.5-ounce) can full-fat coconut milk

1 cup oyster mushrooms, chopped into bite-size pieces

1 teaspoon salt

2 tablespoons Red Boat fish sauce

1 lime, for serving

Cilantro, chopped, for serving

1. On a clean cutting board, trim both ends of the lemongrass to the white, meaty portion of the stalk. Cut lengthwise in half. Cut the ginger in half and then gently smash the ginger and garlic.

2. In a large saucepan over medium heat, combine the lemongrass, ginger, garlic, and lime leaves with the broth. Bring to a gentle boil and reduce the heat to low. Cook for 10 minutes.

3. Using a slotted spoon or mesh spider, remove the large pieces from the broth. Add the chicken pieces to the pan and bring to a gentle boil. Add the coconut milk, mushrooms, salt, and fish sauce. Reduce the heat to low and simmer for 25 minutes.

4. Top each bowl with a squeeze of lime juice and a pinch of cilantro. Enjoy!

SUBSTITUTION TIP: If you cannot find kaffir lime leaves, substitute lime zest and 2 tablespoons of lime juice.

PER SERVING: CALORIES: 527; CARBS: 6G; SUGAR: 2G; FIBER: 1G; FAT: 27G; SATURATED FAT: 18G; PROTEIN: 64G; SODIUM: 1498MG

stewed pork and escarole

DAIRY FREE • PALEO

MAKES 6 SERVINGS This recipe is a spinoff of the traditional Chinese dish, lion's head meatball. Even though this twist on the classic recipe makes it cleanse friendly, it is still full of flavor.

PREP TIME: 10 minutes
COOK TIME: 60 minutes

1½ pounds ground pastured pork

1 egg

1 teaspoon salt

1 teaspoon freshly ground black pepper

2 tablespoons white wine vinegar

¼ cup water chestnuts, chopped

40 ounces Chicken Bone Broth
  (page 30), divided

Arrowroot powder, for dusting

1 tablespoon sesame oil

1 large head escarole, cleaned and
  chopped (9 to 10 cups)

1-inch piece fresh ginger, peeled and sliced

4 baby bok choy, halved

½ teaspoon fish sauce

2 teaspoons coconut aminos

1 scallion, thinly sliced, for serving

1. In a large bowl, combine the pork, egg, salt, pepper, vinegar, water chestnuts, and 3 tablespoons of broth. Stir by hand until mixed well. The meat will be sticky. Form into 2-inch balls, lightly dusting each with arrowroot powder.

2. In a nonstick sauté pan over medium heat, warm the sesame oil. Brown the meatballs in a single layer until seared on all sides, but not cooked through.

3. In a Dutch oven layer half of the escarole on the bottom. Top with the seared meatballs. Cover the meatballs with the remaining escarole. Add the remaining broth, ginger, bok choy, fish sauce, and coconut aminos. Simmer over low heat, covered, for 45 to 60 minutes.

4. Garnish with the scallion and serve.

PER SERVING: CALORIES: 398; CARBS: 5G; SUGAR: 1G; FIBER: 2G; FAT: 28G; SATURATED FAT: 10G; PROTEIN: 31G; SODIUM: 653MG

beet 'n' beef soup

DAIRY FREE • GLUTEN FREE • PALEO

MAKES 4 SERVINGS **Beets are an excellent source of vitamin C, folate, potassium, and manganese. According to Traditional Chinese Medicine teachings, beets are good at "building blood," the life of your body. Not only does this soup taste good, it's also incredibly nourishing.**

PREP TIME: 5 minutes
COOK TIME: 1 hour 5 minutes

4 large beets (about 3 cups cooked beets)
2 tablespoons coconut oil
1 onion, chopped
4 carrots, peeled and cut into coins
2 teaspoons salt
40 ounces Beef Bone Broth (page 32)
Juice and zest of ½ orange

1. Preheat the oven to 375°F.

2. On a clean cutting board, cut off both ends of the beets and wrap the beets in aluminum foil. Place on a baking sheet and roast for 30 minutes. Let cool for 10 minutes. Use the foil to remove the skin from the beets.

3. In a Dutch oven over medium, heat the oil and sauté the onion and carrots for 5 minutes. Stir often.

4. Add the beets, salt, and broth to the Dutch oven. Bring to a gentle boil and then reduce the heat to low. Simmer for 30 minutes.

5. Remove the pan from the heat and let cool slightly. Using an immersion blender, purée the soup until smooth.

6. Add the orange juice and mix well. Serve topped with orange zest.

> PREP TIP: Use gloves or you will have beet-colored fingers. You can also roast the beets ahead of time to cut the cooking time in half.

PER SERVING: CALORIES: 214; CARBS: 23G; SUGAR: 15G; FIBER: 5G; FAT: 7G; SATURATED FAT: 6G; PROTEIN: 16G; SODIUM: 1569MG

tomato soup

DAIRY FREE • GLUTEN FREE • PALEO

MAKES 10 SERVINGS There's nothing quite like creamy tomato soup to cheer you up. It's a classic American dish that's quintessential comfort food. This recipe offers a twist on the tradition by incorporating coconut milk in place of heavy cream and beef bone broth to boost the flavor profile. Even this variation screams comfort any day of the week.

PREP TIME: 5 minutes

COOK TIME: 40 minutes

1 large onion, chopped

3 garlic cloves

2 tablespoons coconut oil

1 teaspoon sea salt

2 large carrots, peeled and sliced

2 (28-ounce) cans whole peeled tomatoes

5 fresh basil leaves

1 (13.5-ounce) can full-fat coconut milk

20 ounces Beef Bone Broth (page 32)

1. In a Dutch oven over medium heat, sauté the onion and garlic in the oil for 5 minutes, stirring frequently. Add the salt.

2. Add the carrots and cook for an additional 5 minutes, stirring frequently.

3. Add the tomatoes, basil, coconut milk, and broth. Bring to a gentle boil and reduce the heat to simmer for 30 minutes.

4. Remove the pan from the heat and let cool slightly. Using an immersion blender, purée the soup until smooth.

PER SERVING: CALORIES: 153; CARBS: 10G; SUGAR: 5G; FIBER: 2G; FAT: 10G; SATURATED FAT: 9G; PROTEIN: 5G; SODIUM: 533MG

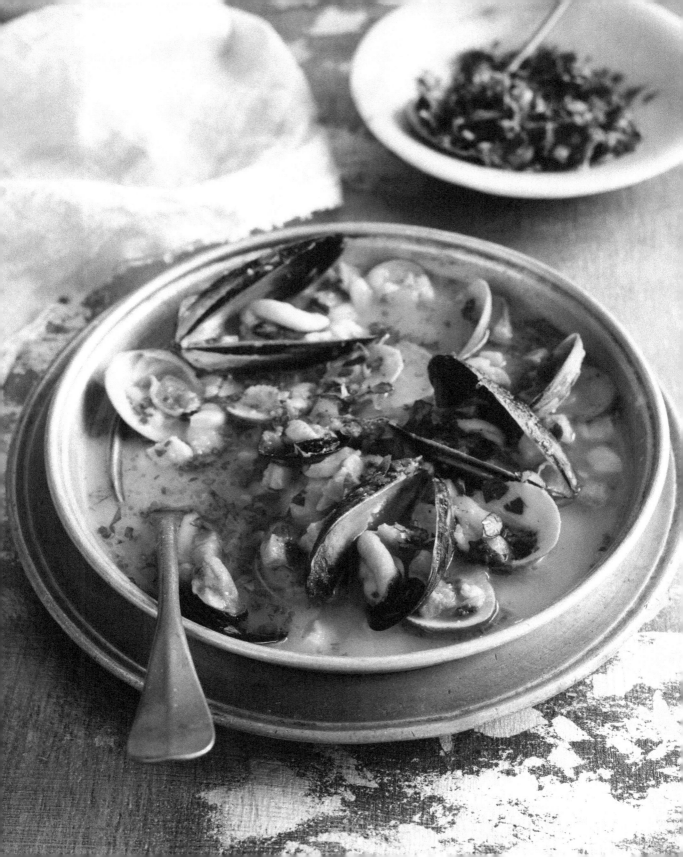

mussel and clam soup
with white beans and gremolata

DAIRY FREE • GLUTEN FREE • PALEO • QUICK & EASY

MAKES 4 SERVINGS You'll be surprised at how quickly and easily this impressive shellfish soup comes together. It starts with rich Chicken Bone Broth (page 30) and gets even richer and more flavorful as the shellfish cooks in it. A dollop of garlicky gremolata adds a bright hit of flavor.

PREP TIME: 10 minutes

COOK TIME: 10 minutes

FOR THE GREMOLATA

½ cup chopped flat-leaf parsley

1 garlic clove, finely minced

2 lemons

FOR THE SOUP

2 tablespoons extra-virgin olive oil or ghee

2 garlic cloves, minced

20 ounces Chicken Bone Broth (page 30)

1½ cups cooked cannellini beans

2 bay leaves

Pinch red pepper flakes

24 mussels, scrubbed and de-bearded

24 clams, scrubbed

Kosher salt

Freshly ground black pepper

TO MAKE THE GREMOLATA

In a small bowl, combine the parsley and garlic. Using a grater or zester, grate the zest of both lemons into the parsley. Toss together with a fork until well combined.

TO MAKE THE SOUP

1. In a Dutch oven, heat the olive oil (or ghee, if using) over medium heat. Add the garlic and cook, stirring, until softened, about 1 minute. Add the broth, beans, bay leaves, and red pepper flakes and bring to a simmer.

2. Add the mussels and clams, cover the pot, and steam until most of the mussels and clams open up, about 10 minutes (discard any that don't open in 10 minutes). Taste and season the broth with salt and pepper as needed.

3. To serve, divide the mussels and clams among four serving bowls and spoon the broth and beans over the top. Dollop each serving with a spoonful of gremolata and serve hot.

PER SERVING: CALORIES: 466; CARBS: 34G; SUGAR: 3G; FIBER: 7G; FAT: 15G; SATURATED FAT: 2G; PROTEIN: 50G; SODIUM: 532MG

thai carrot soup

DAIRY FREE • GLUTEN FREE • PALEO

MAKES 8 SERVINGS If you love carrots, this recipe is a must-try. It's a perfect soup to enjoy on the go because you can easily transport it in an insulated container. The ingredients are simple, but the soup is very flavorful.

PREP TIME: 5 minutes

COOK TIME: 40 minutes

1 large onion, diced

3 garlic cloves

2 tablespoons coconut oil

1 teaspoon sea salt

2 pounds carrots, peeled and cut into
    ½-inch-thick slices

20 ounces Chicken Bone Broth (page 30)

1 (13.5-ounce) can full-fat coconut milk

1 tablespoon red curry paste

1. In a Dutch oven over medium heat, sauté the onion and garlic in oil for 5 minutes, stirring frequently. Add the salt.

2. Add the carrots and cook for an additional 5 minutes, stirring frequently.

3. Add the broth, coconut milk, and curry paste, and bring to a gentle boil. Reduce the heat to low and simmer for 30 minutes.

4. Remove the pan from the heat and let cool slightly. Using an immersion blender, purée the soup until smooth.

PER SERVING: CALORIES: 162; CARBS: 14G; SUGAR: 7G; FIBER: 3G; FAT: 10G; SATURATED FAT: 8G; PROTEIN: 5G; SODIUM: 503MG

broccoli soup

DAIRY FREE • GLUTEN FREE • PALEO

MAKES 8 SERVINGS This is my absolute favorite breakfast soup! It's full of superfoods and keeps me full all morning. The addition of cauliflower makes this soup seem creamy without any dairy, which means that you can enjoy it throughout the cleanse! And it goes well with whichever bone broth you want to use from chapter 4.

PREP TIME: 5 minutes
COOK TIME: 40 minutes

1 large onion, chopped
2 garlic cloves, peeled
2 tablespoons coconut oil
1 pound broccoli, chopped
1 pound cauliflower, chopped
40 ounces bone broth
1 teaspoon sea salt

1. In a Dutch oven over medium heat, sauté the onion and garlic in oil for 5 minutes, stirring frequently.

2. Add the broccoli and cauliflower. Cook for an additional 5 minutes, stirring frequently.

3. Add the broth and salt and bring to a gentle boil. Reduce the heat and simmer for 30 minutes.

4. Remove the pan from the heat and let cool slightly. Using an immersion blender, purée the soup until smooth. Enjoy!

PER SERVING: CALORIES: 99: CARBS: 8G; SUGAR: 3G; FIBER: 3G; FAT: 3G; SATURATED FAT: 0G; PROTEIN: 9G: SODIUM: 380MG

everything but the tortilla chicken soup

DAIRY FREE • GLUTEN FREE • PALEO

MAKES 8 SERVINGS **This is a cleanse-friendly, creamy spin on the classic chicken tortilla soup. I love that I can warm it up in the morning, pour it into an insulated container, and have lunch on the go. It's nutrient dense and packs a punch with all of the peppers.**

PREP TIME: 5 minutes

COOK TIME: 40 minutes

1 red bell pepper

1 green bell pepper

1 jalapeño pepper

2 poblano peppers

1 onion, sliced

2 garlic cloves, unpeeled

1 (28-ounce) can fire-roasted tomatoes

20 ounces Chicken Bone Broth (page 30)

2 tablespoons coconut oil

½ teaspoon ground cumin

1 teaspoon salt

½ teaspoon freshly ground black pepper

1. Preheat the oven to 375 °F.

2. Line a baking sheet with aluminum foil. Place the bell peppers, jalapeño, poblanos, onion, and garlic on the sheet. Roast for 10 minutes, turning the vegetables over once halfway through. Let cool for 5 minutes. Put the poblano peppers into a bowl and cover with plastic wrap to steam.

3. Remove the skin from the poblano peppers. Remove the peel from the garlic. Slice the the peppers, discarding the stems and seeds.

4. Add the peppers, onion, garlic, tomatoes, broth, coconut oil, cumin, salt, and pepper to a Dutch oven. Bring to a gentle boil and reduce the heat to low. Simmer for 30 minutes.

5. Remove the pan from the heat and let cool slightly. Using an immersion blender, purée the soup until smooth. Serve or refrigerate.

PER SERVING: CALORIES: 81; CARBS: 8G; SUGAR: 4G; FIBER: 2G; FAT: 4G; SATURATED FAT: 3G; PROTEIN: 4G; SODIUM: 516MG

thai chicken soup

DAIRY FREE • GLUTEN FREE • PALEO

MAKES 8 SERVINGS **This recipe is a spinoff of the classic chicken noodle soup. By infusing Thai flavors, you can incorporate different seasonings into your weekly routine.**

PREP TIME: 5 minutes

COOK TIME: 35 minutes

2 onions, diced

2 tablespoons coconut oil

1 teaspoon paprika

1 teaspoon turmeric

1 teaspoon salt

40 ounces Chicken Bone Broth (page 30)

2 (13.5-ounce) cans full-fat coconut milk

1 tablespoon fish sauce

¼ teaspoon chopped ginger

1. In a Dutch oven over medium heat, sauté the onions in the oil for 5 minutes, stirring frequently.

2. Add the paprika, turmeric, and salt. Mix well.

3. Add the broth, coconut milk, fish sauce, and ginger, and bring to a gentle boil. Reduce the heat to low and simmer for 30 minutes.

4. Remove the pan from the heat and let cool slightly. Using an immersion blender, purée the soup until smooth. Enjoy!

PER SERVING: CALORIES: 247; CARBS: 6G; SUGAR: 2G; FIBER: 0G; FAT: 22G; SATURATED FAT: 18G; PROTEIN: 7G; SODIUM: 546MG

mushroom soup

DAIRY FREE • GLUTEN FREE • PALEO

MAKES 8 SERVINGS If you love mush-rooms, you'll love this recipe! The earthiness of the mushrooms and the richness of flavor they bring make this a supremely satisfying soup. Mushrooms are known for their superfood healing powers and this is one of the best ways to introduce them into your diet.

PREP TIME: 10 minutes
COOK TIME: 45 minutes

1 onion, chopped

2 garlic cloves, peeled and sliced

2 tablespoons coconut oil

8 cups fresh cremini mushrooms, roughly chopped

1 cup fresh shiitake mushrooms, roughly chopped

1 cup oyster mushrooms, roughly chopped

2 teaspoons sea salt

20 ounces bone broth

1 (13.5-ounce) can full-fat coconut milk

2 tablespoons reishi powder

2 tablespoons fresh thyme

1. In a Dutch oven over medium heat, sauté the onion and garlic in the oil for 5 minutes, stirring frequently.

2. Add the cremini, shiitake, and oyster mushrooms one at a time to allow them to fit. Add the salt. Cook for 10 minutes.

3. Add the broth, coconut milk, reishi powder, and thyme. Bring to a gentle boil. Reduce the heat to low and simmer for 30 minutes.

4. Remove the pan from the heat and let cool slightly. Using an immersion blender, purée until smooth.

PER SERVING: CALORIES: 267; CARBS: 19G; SUGAR: 4G; FIBER: 4G; FAT: 17G; SATURATED FAT: 14G; PROTEIN: 10G; SODIUM: 854MG

french onion soup

GLUTEN FREE • PALEO

MAKES 4 SERVINGS French onion soup is a classic that just needed a little tweak to make it diet friendly. Instead of topping with a crostini and Gruyère, I substituted Parsnip Purée (page 63). The sweetness of the parsnips pairs really well with the saltiness of the soup.

PREP TIME: 5 minutes

COOK TIME: 50 minutes

2 pounds onions, cut into ¼-inch-thick half moons

4 garlic cloves, minced

2 teaspoons sea salt

4 tablespoons ghee

40 ounces Beef Bone Broth (page 32)

1 tablespoon fresh thyme leaves

1 teaspoon red wine vinegar

2 cups Parsnip Purée (page 63)

1. In a Dutch oven over medium heat, sauté the onions, garlic, and salt in the ghee for about 10 minutes.

2. Add the broth, thyme, and vinegar to the pot. Bring to a gentle boil and reduce the heat to low. Simmer for 30 minutes, uncovered.

3. Preheat the oven to 425°F.

4. Ladle the soup into four individual oven-safe bowls and top with the parsnip purée. Roast for 10 minutes.

5. Let cool for 5 minutes before serving. Enjoy!

PER SERVING: CALORIES: 331; CARBS: 34G; SUGAR: 13G; FIBER: 7G; FAT: 16G; SATURATED FAT: 9G; PROTEIN: 16G; SODIUM: 1178MG

creamy pea soup
with avocado and apple salsa

GLUTEN FREE • QUICK & EASY

MAKES 4 SERVINGS Split pea soup gets
a fresh flavor update here with the
addition of a bright and flavorful salsa
made of apples and avocado as well
as a garnish of fresh greens and herbs.
Instead of heavy cream, this soup gets its
richness from full-fat coconut milk.

PREP TIME: 15 minutes
Cook time: 15 minutes

FOR THE SOUP

2 tablespoons ghee

1 tablespoon extra-virgin olive oil

1 large onion, chopped

3 celery stalks, diced

1 white potato, peeled and diced

Kosher salt

3 cups frozen peas, thawed

5 cups Chicken Bone Broth (page 30)

⅔ cup full-fat coconut milk

Freshly ground black pepper

FOR THE SALSA

2 large Granny Smith apples, peeled,
   cored, and diced

1 large ripe avocado, halved, pitted,
   peeled, and diced

Juice of 1 lime

½ teaspoon kosher salt

¼ teaspoon freshly ground black pepper

TO SERVE

Balsamic vinegar

Red pepper flakes

1 large handful arugula leaves

1 handful baby spinach

Several fresh dill sprigs

1 lime, cut into wedges

Extra-virgin olive oil

TO MAKE THE SOUP

1. In a large Dutch oven set over medium heat, melt the ghee with the oil. Add the onion, celery, potato, and a pinch of salt. Cook, stirring frequently, until the vegetables soften, 6 to 8 minutes. Stir in the peas and broth, and bring to a boil. Once boiling, reduce to a gentle simmer and partially cover with a lid.

2. Cook for 5 minutes. Remove about ½ cup of peas before stirring in the coconut milk.

3. Purée the soup with an immersion blender or in a food processor, working in batches as needed.

4. Return the reserved peas to the soup and season with salt and pepper.

TO MAKE THE SALSA

In a mixing bowl, stir together the apples, avocado, lime juice, salt, and pepper.

TO SERVE

Ladle the soup into warm bowls. Drizzle with some balsamic vinegar and top with red pepper flakes, arugula leaves, spinach, dill, lime wedges, the prepared salsa, and a drizzle of extra-virgin olive oil.

PER SERVING: CALORIES: 473; CARBS: 42G; SUGAR: 18G; FIBER: 12G; FAT: 27G; SATURATED FAT: 12G; PROTEIN: 20G; SODIUM: 440MG

paleo pork ramen

DAIRY FREE • PALEO

MAKES 8 SERVINGS This dish takes a little more time to finish, but it is well worth it! I really enjoy making this for guests because it is a gourmet recipe that will impress with its slow-cooked pork and colorful toppings, but won't stress you out with extensive preparation.

PREP TIME: 10 minutes

COOK TIME: 40 minutes, plus 8 hours in slow cooker

2½ pounds pastured pork shoulder

FOR THE SOUP

2 tablespoons ghee

1 tablespoon extra-virgin olive oil

1 large onion, chopped

3 celery stalks, diced

1 white potato, peeled and diced

Kosher salt

3 cups frozen peas, thawed

5 cups Chicken Bone Broth (page 30)

⅔ cup full-fat coconut milk

Freshly ground black pepper

1 tablespoon curry powder

1 acorn squash, peeled and cubed

2 cups cremini mushrooms, sliced

2 tablespoons sesame oil

2 cups zucchini zoodles

4 softboiled eggs

Kosher salt

1 cup chopped carrots

1 jalapeño pepper, sliced

1 scallion, chopped

¼ cup chopped fresh cilantro

1. In a slow cooker, cover the pork with the broth, coconut aminos, vinegar, and fish sauce. Add the curry paste, ginger, chili paste, lime juice, five spice powder, and 1 teaspoon of pepper. Cover the slow cooker and cook on low for 8 hours or high for 6 hours.

2. Preheat the oven to 400°F about 40 minutes prior to eating.

3. In a small bowl, mix together the melted coconut oil, curry powder, and the remaining 1 teaspoon of pepper.

4. On a greased baking sheet, toss together the cubed squash and curry mixture until the squash is well coated. Bake for 30 to 40 minutes, tossing a couple of times during cooking. The squash should be lightly browned and crisp.

5. Meanwhile, remove the pork from the slow cooker and add the mushrooms to the cooker. Cover and crank the heat to high. Lightly shred the pork with two forks.

6. In a large skillet over medium heat, brown some of the pork in the sesame oil. Allow the pork to caramelize, without stirring, for about 2 minutes. Then stir and allow the pork to continue to caramelize, 3 to 5 minutes total. Remove the pork from the skillet and repeat with the remaining pork. Set aside and keep warm.

7. Add the zucchini zoodles to the slow cooker and allow them to cook for about 5 minutes. Once the noodles are cooked, stir in half of the pork.

8. Ladle the soup into bowls. Top with extra caramelized pork, curry-roasted squash, and an egg. Season the egg with salt and pepper. Add the carrots, jalapeño, scallion, and cilantro.

> PREP TIP: If you're looking to shorten the cooking time, make the pork ahead of time.

PER SERVING: CALORIES: 658; CARBS: 15G; SUGAR: 2G; FIBER: 3G; FAT: 46G; SATURATED FAT: 17G; PROTEIN: 45G; SODIUM: 1056MG

pho real soup

DAIRY FREE • PALEO

MAKES 4 TO 6 SERVINGS **This dish reminds me of my dad. I have fond memories of eating the best pho at a hole-in-the-wall restaurant. We would sip the broth and slurp down the noodles. The bone broth was always my favorite.**

PREP TIME: 10 minutes

COOK TIME: 55 minutes

2 onions, quartered

1 (4-inch) piece of ginger, peeled and halved

1 cinnamon stick

1 teaspoon fennel seeds

1 teaspoon coriander seeds

3 star anise pods

6 cloves

20 ounces Beef Bone Broth (page 32)

2 tablespoons fish sauce

2 cups butternut squash zoodles

1 pound sirloin steak, thinly sliced across the grain

TOPPINGS

Fresh Thai basil

Bean sprouts

Thinly sliced red chiles

Lime wedges

Hoisin sauce

1. Turn the broiler to high.

2. On a baking sheet, spread the quartered onions and halved ginger. Broil for 10 to 15 minutes, turning occasionally so they are charred or browned on all sides.

3. In a dry sauté pan over low heat, combine the cinnamon, fennel, coriander, star anise, and cloves. Cook until fragrant, stirring occasionally, about 5 minutes. Remove from the heat and wrap with the cheesecloth to make a small bundle.

4. In a medium saucepan over medium heat, warm the broth with the onion and ginger mixture and the toasted aromatics. Add the fish sauce and bring to a gentle boil, then reduce the heat to low. Simmer for 30 minutes.

5. Remove the seasonings. Add the zoodles and steak. Cook for 5 minutes.

6. Serve topped with all or just your favorite toppings.

PER SERVING: CALORIES: 300; CARBS: 11G; SUGAR: 4G; FIBER: 2G; FAT: 9G; SATURATED FAT: 3G; PROTEIN: 42G; SODIUM: 774MG

sweet potato and lime soup

DAIRY FREE • GLUTEN FREE • PALEO

MAKES 6 SERVINGS **This recipe has a lot of southwestern inspiration. You'll love the boldness and brightness of the ingredients when combined.**

PREP TIME: 10 minutes

COOK TIME: 40 minutes

2 tablespoons coconut oil

1 leek, washed, trimmed, halved lengthwise, and cut into half moons

4 garlic cloves, sliced

1 cup sliced carrots

5 cups roughly chopped sweet potatoes

40 ounces Chicken Bone Broth (page 30) or Beef Bone Broth (page 32)

1 (13.5-ounce) can full-fat coconut milk

2 teaspoons sea salt

1 teaspoon ground cumin

1 teaspoon paprika

Juice of ½ lime

¼ cup chopped cilantro, for garnish (optional)

1. In a large stockpot over medium heat, combine the oil, leek, and garlic. Sauté for 3 minutes, stirring frequently. Add the carrots and sweet potatoes, and cook for an additional 5 minutes.

2. Add the broth, coconut milk, salt, cumin, and paprika. Bring to a gentle boil and reduce the heat to low. Simmer for 30 minutes and then add the lime juice.

3. Remove the pot from the heat and let cool slightly. Using an immersion blender, blend until smooth. Serve garnished with cilantro, if desired.

PER SERVING: CALORIES: 316; CARBS: 30G; SUGAR: 7G; FIBER: 4G; FAT: 17G; SATURATED FAT: 14G; PROTEIN: 11G; SODIUM: 946MG

spiralized carrot noodle soup
with arugula pesto and chicken meatballs

DAIRY FREE • PALEO • QUICK & EASY

MAKES 4 TO 6 SERVINGS This is a far cry
from your grandmother's chicken soup,
but it's even better for your health.
Crisp-tender spiralized carrots stand in
for the traditional wheat noodles. The
chicken meatballs, cherry tomatoes,
and quick arugula pesto give it flavor
without weighing it down.

PREP TIME: 15 minutes
COOK TIME: 20 minutes

FOR THE PESTO

¼ cup toasted pine nuts

1 garlic clove

2 cups (packed) arugula leaves

2 tablespoons freshly squeezed lemon juice

3 tablespoons nutritional yeast

½ tablespoon kosher salt

½ tablespoon extra-virgin olive oil

FOR THE MEATBALLS

1 pound ground pastured chicken

1 egg

2 tablespoons minced onion

1 tablespoon minced garlic

2 teaspoons Worcestershire sauce

1 tablespoon coconut or extra-virgin olive oil

FOR THE SOUP

2 tablespoons extra-virgin olive oil

1 onion, chopped

20 ounces Chicken Bone Broth (page 30)
    or Turkey Bone Broth (page 38)

2 carrots, peeled and spiralized

1 teaspoon salt

1 teaspoon freshly ground black pepper

1 pint cherry tomatoes, halved

1 cup arugula leaves

TO MAKE THE PESTO

In a food processor, combine the pine nuts, garlic, arugula, lemon juice, yeast, and salt and process to a paste. With the processor running, slowly drizzle the oil through the tube into the paste in a steady stream until well combined and smooth.

TO MAKE THE MEATBALLS

1. In a medium mixing bowl, combine the chicken, egg, onion, garlic, and Worcestershire sauce and mix well. Form the mixture into 12 balls.

2. In a large sauté pan over medium heat, heat the oil and cook the meatballs until they are browned on all sides and cooked through, about 10 minutes.

TO MAKE THE SOUP

1. In a Dutch oven over medium-high heat, heat the oil. Add the onion and cook, stirring, until softened, about 5 minutes.

2. Add the broth to the pot and bring to a simmer. Add the carrots, salt, and pepper and simmer for 3 to 4 minutes, until the carrots are just tender.

3. To serve, scoop out the carrots and divide them among serving bowls. Top with some of the tomatoes, meatballs, and arugula. Ladle hot broth over the top and add a spoonful of pesto to each bowl. Serve immediately.

PER SERVING: CALORIES: 476; CARBS: 14G; SUGAR: 4G; FIBER: 4G; FAT: 33G; SATURATED FAT: 8G; PROTEIN: 34G; SODIUM: 1684MG

Ancient Nutrition

Before cooking vessels were invented, many cultures used empty abdominal pouches from slaughtered animals to cook meat, bones, vegetables, herbs, and water. The first earthenware pots were made and used in ancient China (where the first written documentation of Traditional Chinese Medicine began in the second century BCE) and they were used to cook food over low temperatures in fire pits. Not long after this medicine began to be widely used, bone broth was prescribed by medical practitioners. Chinese medicine used bone broth to nourish the kidneys, support the vital essence (Qi), and to build blood. The term "build blood" refers to blood as one's life force. In fact, as long as there was fuel for their fire, nearly every ancestral culture had a pot of broth slowly simmering over the fire as the original "fast food." Unfortunately, during the 1940s and 1950s, in an effort to make more profit for shareholders, companies such as Campbell's replaced their real ingredients with artificial flavors and MSG. So, broths and stocks started to contain nothing more than MSG and flavored water. The modern popularity of bone broth has started to turn the tide. By slowly simmering bones, meat, vegetables, and herbs in water for a long time, you are creating a nutrient-dense elixir that has always had its roots in healing and nourishment.

butternut squash soup

GLUTEN FREE • PALEO

MAKES 8 SERVINGS **At the first sight of leaves falling, I love whipping this soup up. You'll love the sweetness and savory flavors of this soup, and I bet it will become an autumn classic in your home, too.**

PREP TIME: 5 minutes

COOK TIME: 60 minutes

1 (4-pound) butternut squash, halved and seeded

2 teaspoons sea salt, plus more for seasoning squash

Extra-virgin olive oil

1 large onion, diced

1 Granny Smith apple, cored, peeled, and chopped

2 tablespoons ghee

5 fresh sage leaves, chopped

40 ounces Chicken Bone Broth (page 30), Turkey Bone Broth (page 38), or Beef Bone Broth (page 32)

1 cup full-fat coconut milk

¼ cup pepitas (optional)

1. Preheat the oven to 425°F.

2. In a roasting pan, lay the butternut squash halves, cut-side up, and drizzle with salt and olive oil. Roast for 25 minutes, until soft.

3. In a Dutch oven over medium heat, sauté the onion and apple in the ghee for 2 minutes, stirring frequently.

4. Add the sage, broth, salt, and coconut milk. Bring to a gentle boil and reduce the heat to low. Simmer for 30 minutes.

5. Remove the pan from the heat and let cool slightly. Using an immersion blender, blend the soup until smooth. Serve topped with the pepitas (if using).

PER SERVING: CALORIES: 225; CARBS: 30G; SUGAR: 8G; FIBER: 7G; FAT: 10G; SATURATED FAT: 7G; PROTEIN: 8G; SODIUM: 656MG

green garden soup

MAKES 8 SERVINGS Beautifully green and delicious! You'll love this soup whether you love *or* hate green veggies. This is also a great way to get the kids in your life to eat and enjoy eating these greens.

PREP TIME: 10 minutes

COOK TIME: 35 minutes

2 cups chopped broccoli

2 garlic cloves, sliced

2 onions, chopped

3 tablespoons ghee

40 ounces bone broth

1 teaspoon sea salt

1 teaspoon freshly ground black pepper

12 ounces spinach, chopped

1 bunch green chard, chopped

1 tablespoon freshly squeezed lime juice

¼ cup pepitas (optional)

1. In a Dutch oven over medium heat, sauté the broccoli, garlic, and onions in the ghee for 5 minutes, stirring frequently.

2. Add the broth, salt, pepper, spinach, and chard. Bring to a gentle boil and then reduce the heat to low. Simmer for 30 minutes and then add the lime juice.

3. Remove the pan from the heat and let cool slightly. Using an immersion blender, blend until smooth.

4. Top with the pepitas (if using) and enjoy!

PER SERVING: CALORIES: 222; CARBS: 14G; SUGAR: 4G; FIBER: 6G; FAT: 12G; SATURATED FAT: 7G; PROTEIN: 18G; SODIUM: 1122MG

zucchini soup

GLUTEN FREE • PALEO

MAKES 4 SERVINGS **If your garden is producing a ton of zucchini, you can make a few gallons of this soup to freeze and eat throughout the winter. After zucchini bread, this is my favorite way to eat zucchini.**

PREP TIME: 10 minutes

COOK TIME: 50 minutes

1 onion, chopped

2 garlic cloves, thickly sliced

2 tablespoons ghee

4 zucchini, peeled and chopped

1 teaspoon salt

1 teaspoon freshly ground black pepper

¼ cup coconut cream

40 ounces bone broth

¼ teaspoon ground nutmeg (optional)

1. In a Dutch oven, sauté the onion and garlic in the ghee for 3 minutes, stirring frequently.

2. Add the zucchini, salt, pepper, coconut cream, and broth. Bring to a gentle boil and reduce the heat to low. Simmer for 45 minutes.

3. Remove the pan from the heat and let cool slightly. Using an immersion blender, blend the soup until smooth.

4. Top with the nutmeg (if using) and serve.

PER SERVING: CALORIES: 165; CARBS: 11G; SUGAR: 5G; FIBER: 3G; FAT: 8G; SATURATED FAT: 4G; PROTEIN: 15G; SODIUM: 590MG

butternut squash and chicken enchilada soup

GLUTEN FREE • PALEO

MAKES 6 SERVINGS If you enjoy enchiladas, you'll love this soup. It has all of the flavors of enchiladas and is made using only whole foods. Now you can enjoy cleanse-friendly enchiladas in a soup!

PREP TIME: 10 minutes
COOK TIME: 40 minutes

4 garlic cloves, minced

1 onion, chopped

3 tablespoons ghee

1½ cups peeled and cubed butternut squash

5 cups bone broth

2 tablespoons chopped canned chipotle in adobo

1 teaspoon chili powder

1 teaspoon ground cumin

2 grilled chicken breasts, cubed

1 cup chopped scallion

1 (28-ounce) can fire-roasted tomatoes

3 tablespoons tomato paste

Cilantro, for serving

Avocado, for serving

Lime wedges, for serving

1. In a Dutch oven over medium heat, sauté the garlic and onion in the ghee for 3 minutes. Add the butternut squash and cook for 5 minutes, stirring frequently.

2. Add the broth and scrape up any bits stuck to the bottom of the pan. Add the chipotle in adobo, chili powder, and cumin. Stir well.

3. Add the chicken, scallion, tomatoes, and tomato paste. Bring to a gentle boil, reduce the heat, and simmer for 30 minutes.

4. Divide the soup between serving bowls and top with cilantro, avocado, and lime wedges. Enjoy!

PER SERVING: CALORIES: 213; CARBS: 17G; SUGAR: 7G; FIBER: 5G; FAT: 9G; SATURATED FAT: 5G; PROTEIN: 17G; SODIUM: 464MG

kale and apple soup

DAIRY FREE • GLUTEN FREE • PALEO

MAKES 6 SERVINGS **You are not going to believe this is a diet-friendly recipe. The saltiness of the bacon and the sweetness of the apple pair perfectly in this delicious and decadent soup.**

PREP TIME: 5 minutes

COOK TIME: 45 minutes

5 bacon slices

1 onion, chopped

1 apple, cored and chopped

2 garlic cloves, sliced

1 bunch kale, stemmed and chopped

40 ounces bone broth

1 teaspoon sea salt

1 teaspoon freshly ground black pepper

3 tablespoons coconut cream

1. In a Dutch oven over medium heat, cook the bacon, stirring often, until cooked through but not burned, about 3 minutes. Remove the bacon and set aside.

2. In the bacon grease, cook the onion, apple, and garlic for 2 to 3 minutes, stirring frequently.

3. Add the kale, broth, salt, pepper, and coconut cream. Bring to a gentle boil and reduce the heat to low. Simmer for 30 to 40 minutes. Add the bacon in the last 5 minutes of cooking time.

PER SERVING: CALORIES: 95; CARBS: 6G; SUGAR: 3G; FIBER: 1G; FAT: 3G; SATURATED FAT: 0G; PROTEIN: 11G; SODIUM: 508MG

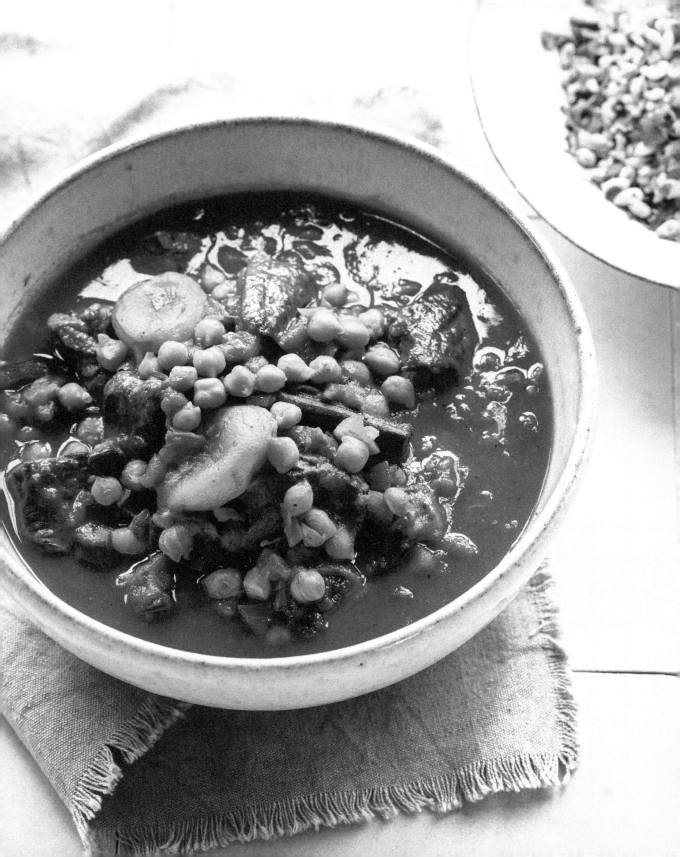

stews

(left) BEEF STEW WITH DRIED APRICOTS AND CHICKPEAS, PAGE 111

roasted poblano beef and pork chili

DAIRY FREE • GLUTEN FREE

MAKES 6 TO 8 SERVINGS Growing up, chili was always one of my favorite dishes. It reminds me of family and sweaters. This roasted poblano beef and pork chili is going to win whatever chili cook-off you enter. It is hearty and delicious with just the right amount of heat, making it perfect for get-togethers! Your guests will be impressed.

PREP TIME: 15 minutes
COOK TIME: 45 minutes

2 jalapeño peppers

1 poblano pepper

1 red bell pepper

1 green bell pepper

4 garlic cloves

1 onion, chopped

1 tablespoon extra-virgin olive oil

1 pound ground pastured pork

1 pound ground grassfed beef

2 teaspoons salt

1 teaspoon freshly ground black pepper

1 teaspoon ground cumin

1 teaspoon paprika

½ teaspoon chili powder

½ teaspoon ground cinnamon

1 teaspoon red pepper flakes

1 cup cooked black beans

1 cup cooked kidney beans

20 ounces Spicy Pork Bone Broth (page 34)

10 ounces Beef Bone Broth (page 32) (add an additional 4 ounces if not using the coffee)

½ cup brewed coffee (optional)

Plantain chips, for serving

Avocado slices for serving

Shredded lettuce, for serving

1. Preheat the oven to 425°F.

2. On a roasting pan, spread the jalapeño peppers, poblano pepper, red bell pepper, and green bell pepper. Roast for 5 minutes, turning once. Add the garlic and roast for a further 5 minutes, turning the peppers another time.

3. Once cooled, skin the garlic by cutting off one end and pushing the garlic flesh through the opening. Put the poblano, red, and green peppers into a bowl, cover with plastic wrap, and leave to rest for a few minutes so they can be peeled easily.

4. In a Dutch oven over medium heat, sauté the onion in the olive oil for 2 minutes, stirring often. Add the pork and beef, breaking the ground meat up with a large wooden spoon. Brown completely.

5. Add the salt, pepper, cumin, paprika, chili powder, cinnamon, and red pepper flakes. Stir to mix well.

6. Peel the peppers, then chop them into bite-size pieces. Mince the garlic.

7. Add the peppers, garlic, black beans, kidney beans, pork broth, and beef broth, and brewed coffee (if using) to the Dutch oven. Bring to a gentle boil and then turn the heat down to low. Simmer for 30 minutes.

8. Top with plantain chips, avocado, or shredded lettuce if you'd like, and serve.

PER SERVING: CALORIES: 574; CARBS: 19G; SUGAR: 3G; FIBER: 5G; FAT: 38G; SATURATED FAT: 14G; PROTEIN: 37G; SODIUM: 870MG

caldo verde with turkey meatballs

DAIRY FREE • PALEO

MAKES 6 SERVINGS This is a spin on the traditional Portuguese soup, caldo verde. The traditional ingredients consist of potatoes, collard greens, olive oil, and salt. I substituted cauliflower and kale in place of the potatoes and collard greens. I really love the way this dish came together with the turkey meatballs. I hope you enjoy it, too!

PREP TIME: 30 minutes
COOK TIME: 1 hour 15 minutes

2 pounds cauliflower florets (about 1 head)

1 teaspoon ground cumin

1 tablespoon smoked paprika

1 teaspoon salt

1 teaspoon freshly ground black pepper

2 tablespoons extra-virgin olive oil

1 pound ground pastured turkey

1 egg

I onion, chopped, plus 2 tablespoons minced

4 garlic cloves, sliced, plus 1 tablespoon minced

2 teaspoons Worcestershire sauce

2 tablespoons coconut oil, divided

1 teaspoon red pepper flakes

8 cups Chicken Bone Broth (page 30)

1 bunch lacinato kale, stemmed and chopped

¼ cup finely chopped fresh parsley

¼ cup finely chopped fresh cilantro

1. Preheat the oven to 450°F.

2. In a large mixing bowl, toss the cauliflower florets with the cumin, smoked paprika, salt, pepper, and olive oil. Place on a baking sheet and roast for 30 minutes.

3. To make the turkey meatballs, in a large bowl, combine the ground turkey, egg, 2 tablespoons of minced onion, 1 tablespoon of minced garlic, and the Worcestershire sauce, and mix together thoroughly. Form into 12 balls.

4. In a Duch oven over medium heat, melt 1 tablespoon of coconut oil and then sear the meatballs on all sides. Set aside. They don't need to be fully cooked, as the soup will cook them through in a later step.

5. Add the remaining 1 tablespoon of coconut oil to the Dutch oven and sauté the chopped onion and sliced garlic for 3 minutes, or until soft. Add the red pepper flakes and mix in for 1 minute. Add the roasted cauliflower and broth. Bring to a gentle boil, then reduce the heat to low.

6. Cook for 30 minutes, slightly covered.

7. Remove the pot from the heat and let cool slightly. Purée the soup with an immersion blender until smooth.

8. Return the pot to the heat and add the meatballs, kale, parsley, and cilantro. Cook for 10 minutes. Season with salt, and serve.

PER SERVING: CALORIES: 325; CARBS: 13G; SUGAR: 4G; FIBER: 4G; FAT: 17G; SATURATED FAT: 7G; PROTEIN: 32G; SODIUM: 653MG

moroccan lamb tagine

DAIRY FREE • GLUTEN FREE • PALEO

MAKES 4 SERVINGS If you're looking for a change of scenery, this is the dish for you! The saltiness of the olives, the sweetness of the apricots, and the richness of the lamb in this dish will mesmerize your mouth. This recipe is perfect for a day when you have a bit more time to cook.

PREP TIME: 10 minutes
COOK TIME: 2 hours 30 minutes

4 pounds boneless lamb shoulder roast, trimmed and cut into 1½-inch pieces

2 teaspoons salt plus ¼ teaspoon

2 teaspoons freshly ground black pepper

3 tablespoons extra-virgin olive oil, divided

1 large onion, halved and cut into ¼-inch-thick slices

1 lemon rind, cut into 4 pieces

1 tablespoon plus 2 teaspoons minced garlic

2½ teaspoons paprika

1 teaspoon ground cumin

½ teaspoon powdered ginger

½ teaspoon ground coriander

½ teaspoon ground cinnamon

¼ teaspoon cayenne pepper

¼ cup cassava flour

5 cups Chicken Bone Broth (page 30)

2 tablespoons honey

1 pound carrots, peeled and cut into 1-inch chunks

1 cup pitted Greek green olives, halved

1 cup dried apricots, chopped

¼ cup minced fresh cilantro

½ teaspoon grated lemon zest

¼ cup freshly squeezed lemon juice

1. Preheat the oven to 325°F.

2. Pat the lamb dry with paper towels and season with 2 teaspoons each of salt and pepper. In a Dutch oven over medium heat, heat 1 tablespoon of oil. Sear the lamb on all sides and then transfer to a bowl. Repeat with 1 tablespoon of oil and the remaining lamb if necessary.

3. Add 1 tablespoon of oil to the Dutch oven. Add the onion, lemon rind, and the remaining ¼ teaspoon of salt. Cook until the onion is softened, stirring often. Stir in the garlic, paprika, cumin, ginger, coriander, cinnamon, and cayenne pepper, and cook until fragrant, about 1 minute. Stir in the flour and cook for 1 minute, stirring until completely mixed.

4. Slowly stir in the broth, scraping the sides of the pot until the bone broth has completely dissolved. Stir in the honey, browned lamb, and any juices in the bowl. Bring to a simmer. Cover, place in the oven, and cook for 1 hour.

5. After an hour, add the carrots, replace the lid, and continue to cook in the oven until the lamb is tender, about 60 to 90 minutes longer.

6. Remove the tagine from the oven and discard the lemon zest strips. Stir in the olives and apricots, cover, and let stand off the heat for 5 minutes. Stir in the cilantro, lemon zest, and lemon juice. Season with salt and pepper.

PER SERVING: CALORIES: 1393; CARBS: 64G; SUGAR: 34G; FIBER: 7G; FAT: 74G; SATURATED FAT: 27G; PROTEIN: 127G; SODIUM: 2080MG

Complementary Diets

If you're interested in just incorporating bone broth into your daily routine, you should consider a paleo, ketogenic, or Whole30 diet. Sipping broth on its own will not protect you from the effects of a high-sugar, processed food-heavy diet, but using a bone broth diet in conjunction with the following diets can work toward meeting your health objectives.

PALEO: On this diet you can only consume the foods that were available in the Paleolithic era. You can eat food like lean meat, fruits, vegetables, seafood, nuts, seeds, and healthy fats. You should avoid dairy, grains, processed food, sugars, legumes, starches, and alcohol. Bone broth is a perfect addition to this diet because it uses the whole animal, much as our ancestors did.

KETOGENIC: This diet focuses on high fat, low carbohydrate intake. The typical caloric ratio is 65 to 75 percent of your calories from fat, 15 to 30 percent of your calories from protein, and only 5 to 10 percent of your calories from carbohydrates. Bone broth is a great addition to this diet because it's low carbohydrate and high protein, making it a perfect meal or snack, especially if you add healthy fats to it.

WHOLE30: Whole30 is a monthlong diet with a paleo focus that removes all processed foods, sugars, grains, and dairy. Bone broth is an excellent vehicle for soups and stews to expand your meal selection throughout the 30-day cleanse.

orange and olive pork stew

DAIRY FREE • GLUTEN FREE • PALEO

MAKES 6 TO 8 SERVINGS Oranges and olives pair nicely in this stew. I love how simple the ingredients are, but how flavorful the dish is when it comes together.

PREP TIME: 10 minutes
COOK TIME: 1 hour

3 pounds pork shoulder, cut into 1-inch pieces

2 tablespoons coconut oil or ghee

1 onion, diced

2 celery stalks, diced

2 carrots, peeled and diced

1 fennel bulb, sliced, fronds reserved

20 ounces Chicken Bone Broth (page 30)

¼ cup white wine vinegar

Juice and zest of 2 oranges

1 cup green olives, pitted and halved

1 teaspoon salt

1 teaspoon freshly ground black pepper

1. In a Dutch oven over medium-high heat, brown the cubed pork in the oil, in batches if necessary, to avoid overcrowding the pot. Remove from the pot when browned, and set aside.

2. In the same pot, sauté the onion, celery, and carrots for about 5 minutes, stirring frequently. Add the fennel and cook for an additional few minutes.

3. Add the broth, vinegar, and browned pork to the pot. Bring to a gentle boil. Add the orange juice. Reduce the heat to low and simmer for 45 minutes. Add the olives and stir well.

4. Top with the reserved fennel fronds and the orange zest. Season with salt and pepper, and serve.

PER SERVING: CALORIES: 889; CARBS: 14G; SUGAR: 3G; FIBER: 3G; FAT: 65G; SATURATED FAT: 24G; PROTEIN: 58G; SODIUM: 1021MG

caldo de pollo

GLUTEN FREE • PALEO

MAKES 6 SERVINGS Literally translated into "soup of chicken," this Mexican chicken soup is hearty and flavorful. The chicken thighs pair perfectly with the richness of the soup and you'll be wishing there was another pot of this soup hiding somewhere after you have finished the first.

PREP TIME: 5 minutes, plus 30 minutes to marinate

COOK TIME: 45 minutes

6 boneless pastured chicken thighs

1 tablespoon extra-virgin olive oil

1 teaspoon garlic salt

1 onion, chopped

2 tablespoons ghee

4 garlic cloves, minced

2 jalapeño peppers, seeded and sliced

1 teaspoon ground cumin

1 teaspoon salt

1 teaspoon freshly ground black pepper

½ teaspoon smoked paprika

½ teaspoon chili powder

½ teaspoon red pepper flakes

1 (28-ounce) can fire-roasted tomatoes

40 ounces Chicken Bone Broth (page 30)

1. In a large bowl, marinate the chicken thighs in the olive oil and garlic salt for 30 minutes on your counter or overnight in your refrigerator.

2. In a medium sauté pan over medium heat, sauté the onion in the ghee for 3 minutes. Add the garlic and jalapeño peppers and cook for an additional 2 minutes, stirring frequently. Add the marinated chicken thighs. Cook for 5 minutes on each side.

3. Add the cumin, salt, pepper, paprika, chili powder, red pepper flakes, tomatoes, and broth. Bring to a gentle boil and reduce the heat to low. Simmer for 30 minutes.

4. Shred the chicken thighs with two forks, and stir to incorporate. Serve immediately.

PER SERVING: CALORIES: 305; CARBS: 11G; SUGAR: 5G; FIBER: 3G; FAT: 15G; SATURATED FAT: 5G; PROTEIN: 30G; SODIUM: 1126MG

chicken and coconut with vegetables

DAIRY FREE • GLUTEN FREE • PALEO

MAKES 4 SERVINGS This is a combination of chicken soup and vegetable soup. The carrots, broccoli, and parsnips pair perfectly with the creamy chicken. This is an excellent way to boost your vegetable intake!

PREP TIME: 10 minutes

COOK TIME: 50 minutes

2 pounds boneless, skinless pastured
    chicken breasts

2 tablespoons coconut oil

1 (13.5-ounce) can full-fat coconut milk

20 ounces Chicken Bone Broth (page 30)

1 cup diced carrots

1 cup broccoli florets, cut into
    bite-size pieces

1 cup diced parsnips

1 teaspoon sea salt

1 teaspoon curry powder

¼ teaspoon ground ginger

¼ teaspoon cayenne pepper

4 tablespoons coconut cream, for serving

Juice of ½ lime, for serving

1. In a Dutch oven over medium heat, cook the chicken breasts in the oil for 6 to 8 minutes per side. Set aside.

2. Add the coconut milk, broth, carrots, broccoli, parsnips, salt, curry powder, ginger, and cayenne to the pot. Bring to a gentle boil and reduce the heat to low. Simmer for 30 minutes. Use two forks to shred the chicken, and add it to the soup.

3. Serve topped with the coconut cream and lime juice.

PER SERVING: CALORIES: 632; CARBS: 16G; SUGAR: 5G; FIBER: 3G; FAT: 37G; SATURATED FAT: 27G; PROTEIN: 59G; SODIUM: 779MG

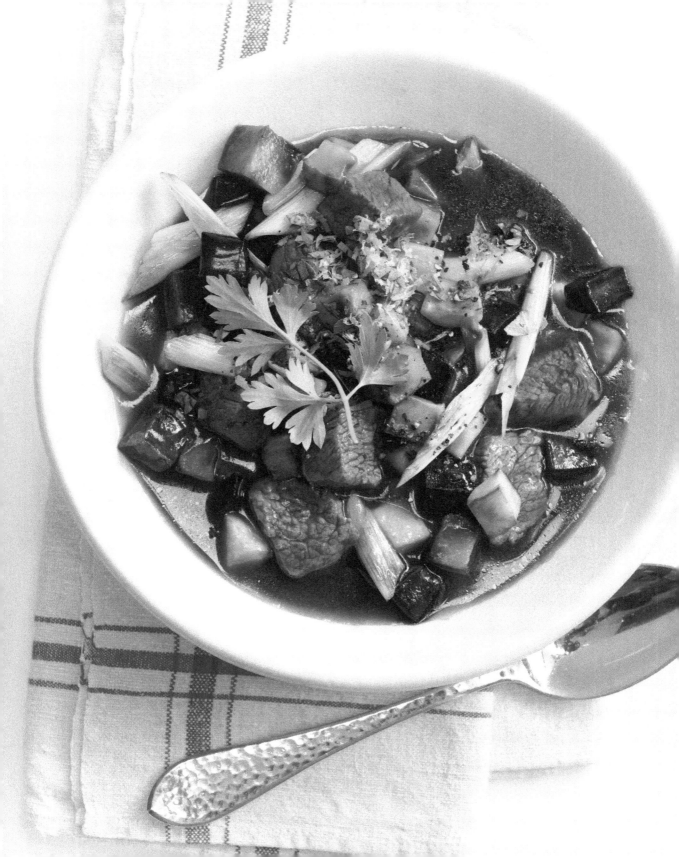

classic beef stew

GLUTEN FREE

MAKES 8 SERVINGS Growing up, I would often ask my mom what we were having for dinner the second I woke up. I have always loved food! If my mom told me we would be having pot roast, I would cry. This classic beef stew is my favorite way to eat pot roast these days. And don't worry, I definitely don't cry about it anymore.

PREP TIME: 10 minutes

COOK TIME: 1 hour 15 minutes

2 pounds boneless chuck roast, cut into 2-inch chunks

2 tablespoons ghee

1 large onion, chopped

2 garlic cloves, sliced

2½ cups (1-inch pieces) carrots

1 potato, cut into 1-inch pieces (about 1 cup)

1 (13.5-ounce) can fire-roasted tomatoes

20 ounces Beef Bone Broth (page 32)

1 tablespoon dried parsley flakes

1 teaspoon fresh thyme leaves

1 teaspoon sea salt

1 teaspoon freshly ground black pepper

1 bay leaf

1. Preheat the oven to 350°F.

2. In a cast iron pot over medium heat, brown the chuck roast in the ghee, about 1 minute per side. Make sure each side is browned, but the pieces do not have to be cooked through. Set aside.

3. Add the onion and garlic and cook for 3 minutes, stirring frequently. Add the carrots and potato and cook for an additional 5 minutes, stirring frequently.

4. Add the tomatoes, broth, parsley, thyme, salt, pepper, and bay leaf. Stir in the browned beef. Bake in the oven for 1 hour, covered.

5. Remove and stir well before serving.

PER SERVING: CALORIES: 346; CARBS: 12G; SUGAR: 4G; FIBER: 3G; FAT: 13G; SATURATED FAT: 6G; PROTEIN: 39G; SODIUM: 520MG

winter vegetable stew

GLUTEN FREE • PALEO

MAKES 6 SERVINGS This soup is as robust as a salad but comes in a delectable bowl of nourishing bone broth. It is incredibly warming and perfect to nourish your body during the winter months.

PREP TIME: 10 minutes
COOK TIME: 40 minutes

1 onion, chopped

6 garlic cloves, sliced

2 tablespoons ghee

2 cups peeled butternut squash, cut into 1-inch chunks

1 cup peeled parsnips, cut into 1-inch chunks

1 cup peeled carrots, cut into 1-inch chunks

1 cup cremini mushrooms, sliced

1 teaspoon salt

2 celery stalks, chopped

40 ounces bone broth

1 can whole peeled tomatoes

1 cup kale, stemmed and chopped

1 teaspoon freshly ground black pepper

1. In a Dutch oven over medium heat, sauté the onion and garlic in the ghee for 3 minutes, stirring frequently.

2. Add the butternut squash, parsnips, carrots, cremini mushrooms, and salt. Cook and stir for 5 minutes.

3. Add the celery, broth, tomatoes, kale, and pepper, and bring to a gentle boil. Reduce the heat to low and simmer for 30 minutes. Serve and enjoy!

PER SERVING: CALORIES: 173; CARBS: 22G; SUGAR: 7G; FIBER: 5G; FAT: 5G; SATURATED FAT: 3G; PROTEIN: 11G; SODIUM: 550MG

beef stew
with dried apricots and chickpeas

GLUTEN FREE

MAKES 6 SERVINGS Adding chickpeas, dried apricots, and cumin gives this beef stew a decidedly North African twist. The apricots add a welcome undercurrent of sweetness to the spicy broth. Serve it with Cauliflower Rice (page 59) for a satisfying meal on a cold winter's evening.

PREP TIME: 10 minutes

COOK TIME: 1 hour 15 minutes

1½ pounds boneless grassfed chuck roast, cut into 2-inch chunks

1 tablespoon ground cumin

1 teaspoon paprika

¼ teaspoon cayenne pepper

Kosher salt

Freshly ground black pepper

2 tablespoons ghee

1 onion, diced

2 garlic cloves, minced

20 ounces Beef Bone Broth (page 32)

2 cups cooked chickpeas

1 (14-ounce) can diced tomatoes

1 (14-ounce) can tomato sauce

8 to 10 dried apricots, thinly sliced

2 tablespoons chopped fresh cilantro or parsley

1. Preheat the oven to 350°F.

2. In a large mixing bowl, toss the beef with the cumin, paprika, cayenne, and a hearty pinch of salt and pepper until the meat is evenly coated.

3. In a Dutch oven over medium-high heat, heat the ghee. Add the beef and cook, stirring occasionally, until it is browned on all sides, 4 to 6 minutes. Remove the beef from the pot and set it aside in a bowl.

4. Add the onion and garlic to the pot and cook, stirring, until softened, about 5 minutes. Return the beef to the pot, along with any accumulated juices, then stir in the broth, chickpeas, diced tomatoes, tomato sauce, and dried apricots. Bring the mixture to a boil, cover, and transfer to the oven.

5. Let the stew cook in the oven for about 1 hour. Serve hot.

PER SERVING: CALORIES: 491; CARBS: 37G; SUGAR: 17G; FIBER: 7G; FAT: 16G; SATURATED FAT: 7G; PROTEIN: 46G; SODIUM: 621MG

irish cabbage stew

DAIRY FREE • GLUTEN FREE • PALEO

MAKES 4 SERVINGS Boiled bacon and cabbage is an Irish staple. The cabbage is full of dietary fiber and a great source of vitamins C, K, and B$_6$. Here we have a diet-friendly version that's just as tasty.

PREP TIME: 5 minutes

COOK TIME: 35 minutes

5 bacon slices, cut into ½-inch pieces

1 onion, chopped

1 garlic clove, sliced

1 cup shredded carrots

20 ounces Spicy Pork Bone Broth (page 34) or Chicken Bone Broth (page 30)

1 teaspoon salt

1 teaspoon freshly ground black pepper

1 small head cabbage, chopped into 1-inch pieces, divided

1. In a Dutch oven over medium-high heat, add the bacon and cook for a few minutes, stirring often so it doesn't burn. Set aside.

2. In the bacon grease, cook the onion and garlic for 2 minutes, stirring frequently.

3. Add the carrots, broth, salt, pepper, and half of the cabbage. Bring to a gentle boil and reduce the heat to a low simmer. At this point, there should be room to add the remaining cabbage to the pot. Add it and cook for 30 minutes, returning the bacon to the pot for the last 5 minutes.

ADD IN: To make this dish more traditional, add two diced Yukon Gold potatoes at the beginning of the recipe and cook until soft.

PER SERVING: CALORIES: 147; CARBS: 16G; SUGAR: 9G; FIBER: 6G; FAT: 5G; SATURATED FAT: 0G; PROTEIN: 12G; SODIUM: 802MG

thai beef stew

MAKES 8 SERVINGS You'll be pleasantly amazed that you created this soul-satisfying dish in your own home. The green beans and zucchini are incredibly appetizing smothered in chile pepper, garlic, and curry.

PREP TIME: 10 minutes

COOK TIME: 40 minutes

1 cup cremini mushrooms, sliced

2 tablespoons red curry paste

2 tablespoons chopped garlic

2 tablespoons coconut oil

1 pound ground grassfed beef

40 ounces Beef Bone Broth (page 32)

1 cup (bite-size pieces) green beans

2 zucchini, halved and cut into ½-inch half moons

Juice of ½ lime

3 tablespoons fish sauce

1 teaspoon coconut aminos

2 tablespoons basil, chopped

2 tablespoons chili garlic sauce

1. In a Dutch oven over medium heat, sauté the mushrooms, curry paste, and garlic in the oil for 3 minutes, stirring frequently. Add the ground beef, using a large spoon to break it into chunks.

2. Add the broth, green beans, zucchini, lime juice, fish sauce, and coconut aminos. Bring to a gentle boil and reduce the heat to low. Simmer for 30 minutes.

3. Add the basil and chili garlic sauce and stir well. Serve and enjoy!

PER SERVING: CALORIES: 217; CARBS: 6G; SUGAR: 2G; FIBER: 1G; FAT: 13G; SATURATED FAT: 7G; PROTEIN: 19G; SODIUM: 806MG

african peanut stew

GLUTEN FREE • PALEO

MAKES 4 SERVINGS This stew is a simple recipe. But don't let that fool you—it has complex flavors. This paleo-friendly recipe is based on a traditional African dish. Feel free to substitute the peanut butter with cashew butter for a lighter dish. You can also substitute Spicy Pork Bone Broth (page 34) for an extra spice kick.

PREP TIME: 10 minutes
COOK TIME: 40 minutes

2 tablespoons ghee

1 red onion, chopped

6 garlic cloves, minced

1 (1-inch) piece fresh ginger, peeled and minced

1 pound boneless pastured chicken thighs, cut into 1-inch chunks

6 cups bone broth

1 cup sliced carrots

1 teaspoon turmeric

1 teaspoon sea salt

½ teaspoon red pepper flakes

6 cups stemmed and chopped collard greens

½ cup peanut butter

½ cup tomato paste

½ cup peanuts (optional)

1. In a Dutch oven over medium heat, heat the ghee. Cook the onion, garlic, and ginger in the ghee for 3 minutes, stirring frequently.

2. Add the chicken and cook for 5 minutes or until it is seared on all sides.

3. Add the broth, carrots, turmeric, salt, and red pepper flakes. Bring to a gentle boil, then reduce the heat to low. Add the collard greens, peanut butter, and tomato paste. Mix well and simmer for 30 minutes.

4. Top with the peanuts (if using) and serve.

PER SERVING: CALORIES: 531; CARBS: 23G; SUGAR: 10G; FIBER: 7G; FAT: 31G; SATURATED FAT: 10G; PROTEIN: 48G; SODIUM: 1096MG

beef stew with beets and parsnips

GLUTEN FREE • PALEO

MAKES 6 SERVINGS Another twist on the classic beef stew, this one includes beets and parsnips, giving it an Eastern European flair. It's like a chunky, meaty version of a classic beet borscht. It's a warming and healing meal that will become a go-to during the winter cold and flu season.

PREP TIME: 10 minutes
COOK TIME: 1 hour 15 minutes

2 tablespoons ghee

1½ pounds boneless grassfed chuck roast, cut into 2-inch chunks

1 onion, diced

2 garlic cloves, minced

2 celery stalks, diced

2 parsnips, peeled and diced

2 beets, peeled and diced

20 ounces Beef Bone Broth (page 32)

¾ teaspoon sea salt

½ teaspoon freshly ground black pepper

1 bay leaf

¼ cup minced flat-leaf parsley, for serving

1. Preheat the oven to 350°F.

2. In a Dutch oven over medium-high heat, heat the ghee. Add the beef and cook, stirring, until it is browned on all sides, 4 to 6 minutes. Remove the beef from the pot and set aside in a bowl.

3. Add the onion and garlic to the pot and cook, stirring frequently, until softened, about 5 minutes. Add the celery, parsnips, and beets and cook, stirring occasionally, for about 5 more minutes.

4. Return the beef to the pot, along with any accumulated juices, and add the broth, salt, pepper, and bay leaf. Cover the pot and transfer to the oven to bake for 1 hour. Serve hot, garnished with the parsley.

PER SERVING: CALORIES: 370; CARBS: 15G; SUGAR: 6G; FIBER: 3G; FAT: 15G; SATURATED FAT: 7G; PROTEIN: 40G; SODIUM: 401MG

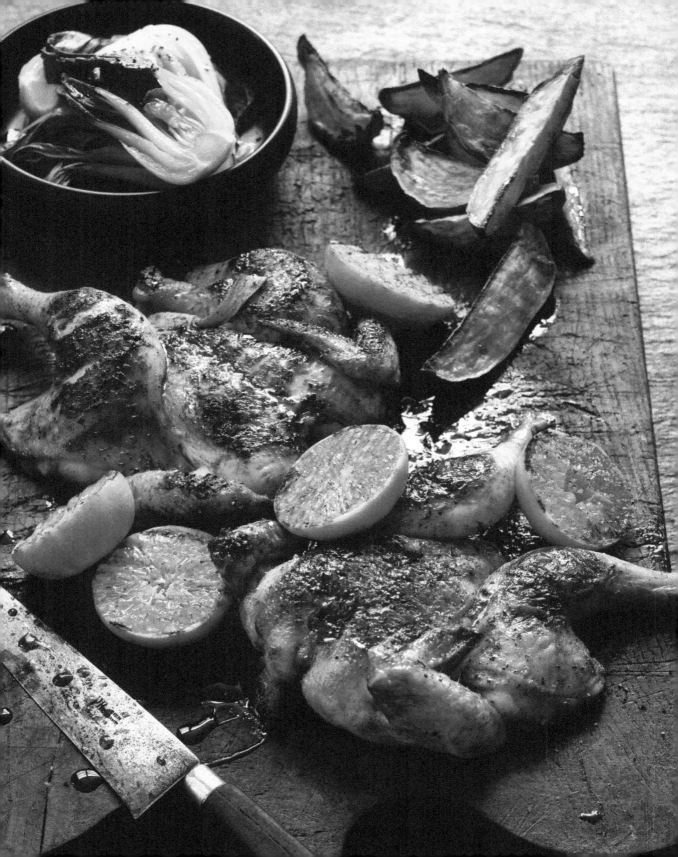

CHAPTER NINE
entrées

(left) ROASTED SPATCHCOCKED CHICKEN, PAGE 135

cajun beef brisket with cherries

DAIRY FREE • PALEO

MAKES 10 SERVINGS If you love sweet, spicy, and savory all in one bite, this is the perfect dish for you! I love that I can use it throughout the week to top salads or tacos, although it's just as good all by itself.

PREP TIME: 10 minutes

COOK TIME: 7 hours in a slow cooker or 2 hours in a pressure cooker

4 pounds grassfed beef brisket

4 tablespoons Cajun seasoning

1 tablespoon beef fat

1 red onion, diced

1 jalapeño pepper, seeded and sliced

1 red bell pepper, seeded and chopped

1 cup frozen cherries

1 tablespoon red pepper flakes

1 teaspoon fish sauce

1 (13.5-ounce) can fire-roasted tomatoes

10 ounces Beef Bone Broth (page 32)

Season the beef brisket liberally with the Cajun seasoning. In a cast-iron pan over high heat, sear each side of the brisket in the beef tallow until browned.

TO COOK:

1. If using a slow cooker, place the seared brisket in the cooker and top with the remaining ingredients. Set for 6 to 7 hours on high heat.

2. If using a pressure cooker, place the seared brisket in the cooker and top with the remaining ingredients. Set on high pressure for 100 minutes.

3. Once finished, shred the beef in the pot directly. Voila!

PREP TIP: If you want, you can make your own Cajun seasoning:

2 teaspoons salt
2 teaspoons paprika
1 teaspoon onion powder
1 teaspoon garlic powder
1 teaspoon chili powder
1 teaspoon white pepper
1 teaspoon dried thyme
1 teaspoon freshly ground black pepper
1 teaspoon dried oregano

Mix together well to combine and store in an airtight container in your spice cabinet.

PER SERVING: CALORIES: 153; CARBS: 6G; SUGAR: 4G; FIBER: 1G; FAT: 7G; SATURATED FAT: 3G; PROTEIN: 16G; SODIUM: 176MG

smothered cremini mushrooms with homestyle brat sausage

GLUTEN FREE • PALEO • QUICK & EASY

MAKES 4 SERVINGS When I first created this dish, I had a room full of people who doubted that it would taste good. But all the bowls were licked clean. This excellent, rich dish is sure to please your crowd.

PREP TIME: 10 minutes

COOK TIME: 20 minutes

1 onion, diced

1 garlic clove, sliced

2 tablespoons ghee, divided

4 bratwursts, split and casings removed

1 cup cremini mushrooms, chopped

1 cup butternut squash zoodles

1 tablespoon fresh thyme leaves

10 ounces Spicy Pork Bone Broth (page 34)

1. In a sauté pan over medium heat, sauté the onion and garlic in 1 tablespoon of ghee for 3 minutes, stirring often, until the onion becomes translucent. Add the bratwurst to the pan. Cook until browned, about 8 minutes.

2. Add the mushrooms and zoodles to the pan. Cook for 3 minutes, until the mushrooms soften.

3. Add the thyme, broth, and the remaining 1 tablespoon of ghee. Cook for 5 minutes. Serve!

SUBSTITUTION TIP: If you don't have access to fresh bratwurst, you can substitute another sausage you like. Just make sure you can remove the casing.

PER SERVING: CALORIES: 387; CARBS: 8G; SUGAR: 2G; FIBER: 1G; FAT: 32G; SATURATED FAT: 13G; PROTEIN: 16G; SODIUM: 722MG

brisket and plantain casserole

DAIRY FREE • GLUTEN FREE • PALEO

MAKES 6 SERVINGS Let me guess . . . you made enough Cajun Beef Brisket with Cherries (page 118) to last a lifetime and you're looking for something new to use those leftovers? This casserole is an excellent option. Plus, it combines other leftovers, is easy to make ahead, and should leave you with plenty of casserole for lunch the next day.

PREP TIME: 20 minutes

COOK TIME: 45 minutes

2 yellow plantains, peeled and cut into strips

1 tablespoon coconut oil

4 cups Cajun Beef Brisket with Cherries (page 118)

2 cups Sweet Potato Purée (page 62)

1. Preheat the oven to 375°F.

2. In a sauté pan over medium heat, sauté the plantains in the oil until lightly browned on both sides, about 10 minutes.

3. In a 9-by-13-inch baking dish, assemble the casserole by layering the bottom of the dish with the plantains. Next, add the beef brisket and top with the sweet potato purée.

4. Cook for 35 minutes. Let cool for 5 minutes and serve.

PER SERVING: CALORIES: 250; CARBS: 35G; SUGAR: 4G; FIBER: 3G; FAT: 7G; SATURATED FAT: 4G; PROTEIN: 12G; SODIUM: 141MG

bone broth burgers

DAIRY FREE • GLUTEN FREE • PALEO • QUICK & EASY

MAKES 8 SERVINGS Burgers are the ultimate comfort food! Good thing this comfort food is also cleanse friendly. I also love turning these burgers into a salad the next day. Just add veggies and dressing with the chopped-up patty. Yum!

PREP TIME: 5 minutes
COOK TIME: 20 minutes

1 pound ground grassfed beef

½ pound ground pastured pork

¾ cup Beef Bone Broth (page 32)

1 teaspoon garlic powder

½ teaspoon cayenne powder

2 tablespoons coconut oil

4 teaspoons salt

4 teaspoons freshly ground black pepper

8 green leaf lettuce leaves

1. In a large bowl, mix together the ground beef, ground pork, bone broth, garlic powder, and cayenne. Form 8 patties.

2. Preheat a sauté pan to high heat and add the oil. Season the outside of the burgers liberally with the salt and pepper. Cook to desired level of doneness.

3. Serve in the lettuce leaves.

ADD IN: Sauté onions in ghee and serve with sauerkraut for the perfect gut-healing recipe.

PER SERVING: CALORIES: 231; CARBS: 0G; SUGAR: 0G; FIBER: 0G; FAT: 18G; SATURATED FAT: 9G; PROTEIN: 16G; SODIUM: 1207MG

paleo shepherd's pie

GLUTEN FREE • PALEO

MAKES 8 SERVINGS This dish is a nutritional powerhouse. And talk about convenient! If you're running short on time, you can make this one ahead and store it in the refrigerator, covered, until you're ready to cook.

PREP TIME: 15 minutes
COOK TIME: 1 hour 10 minutes

6 large sweet potatoes, peeled and roughly chopped
20 ounces Beef Bone Broth (page 32)
3 tablespoons ghee, divided
2 teaspoons salt, divided
1 red onion, chopped
1 garlic clove, sliced
2 pounds ground grassfed beef
1 tablespoon fresh thyme leaves
1 teaspoon smoked paprika
1 teaspoon onion powder
1 cup shredded carrots
1 bunch lacinato kale, stemmed and chopped
1½ cups peas, frozen
Freshly ground black pepper

1. Preheat the oven to 400°F.

2. In a large pot over high heat, bring water to a boil. Cook the sweet potatoes until they are soft enough to be pierced with a fork, about 10 minutes. Drain the water.

3. Add the broth to the pot. Mash the sweet potatoes and broth together with 2 tablespoons of ghee and season with 1 teaspoon of salt. Set aside.

4. Meanwhile, in a sauté pan over medium heat, sauté the onion and garlic in the remaining 1 tablespoon of ghee until soft, about 5 minutes. Add the ground beef and cook until browned, 7 to 10 minutes. Add the fresh thyme, paprika, and onion powder.

5. Next, add the carrots and kale. Simmer, constantly stirring, for 5 minutes. Add the frozen peas.

6. In a 9-by-13-inch baking dish, evenly spread the ground beef mixture. Top with the mashed sweet potatoes. Cover with aluminum foil and bake for 20 minutes.

7. Remove the foil and bake for an additional 20 minutes. Let cool for 10 minutes. Enjoy!

PER SERVING: CALORIES: 403; CARBS: 36G; SUGAR: 7G; FIBER: 5G; FAT: 6G; SATURATED FAT: 14G; PROTEIN: 29G; SODIUM: 719MG

paleo pork tacos

DAIRY FREE • GLUTEN FREE • PALEO

MAKES 6 TO 8 SERVINGS This recipe for pork paleo tacos often makes it into my weekly rotation. It's easy but it will seem gourmet to your friends and family. Plus, it is great as an hors d'oeuvre if necessary.

PREP TIME: 10 minutes

COOK TIME: 30 minutes, plus 6 to 10 hours to roast

4 pounds pastured pork shoulder

1 tablespoon salt, plus 1 teaspoon, divided

1 tablespoon freshly ground black pepper, plus 1 teaspoon, divided

1 tablespoon dried oregano

2 teaspoons ground cumin

2 tablespoons extra-virgin olive oil

1 onion, diced

1 jalapeño pepper, seeded and chopped

4 garlic cloves, sliced

Juice of 1 orange

1 tablespoon red pepper flakes

20 ounces Spicy Pork Bone Broth (page 34)

2 sweet potatoes, cut into ¼-inch-thick slices

1 tablespoon coconut oil

1 red onion, finely chopped

1 scallion, sliced

1. Rinse and dry the pork shoulder, and rub with 1 tablespoon each of salt and pepper. Next, in a small bowl, combine the oregano, cumin, and olive oil. Rub this mixture evenly over the pork.

2. Place the pork in the slow cooker (fatty-side up), and top with the onion, jalapeño, garlic, orange juice, red pepper flakes, and bone broth. Cook on low for 8 to 10 hours or on high for 6 hours.

3. Heat the oven to 350°F.

4. Rub the sweet potato slices with the coconut oil and season lightly with the remaining salt and pepper. Bake for 12 minutes until just browned.

5. The meat should now be tender and falling off the bone. Remove from the slow cooker and let cool slightly. Then shred the pork using two forks.

6. In a large sauté pan over medium heat, sauté the shredded pork until crispy, stirring often. Meanwhile, in a small saucepan over medium-low heat, reduce the pork juices to use as gravy.

7. Layer sweet potatoes and pork to create an open-faced taco, garnish with the red onion and scallion, and enjoy!

PER SERVING: CALORIES: 622; CARBS: 20G; SUGAR: 6G; FIBER: 3G; FAT: 31G; SATURATED FAT: 11G; PROTEIN: 64G; SODIUM: 3042MG

braised short ribs

DAIRY FREE • GLUTEN FREE • PALEO

MAKES 6 SERVINGS This recipe for braised short ribs requires a little more diligence and should be reserved for the weekend or a day when you'll be able to spend time on preparation. But these ribs are definitely worth the extra effort!

PREP TIME: 20 minutes, plus overnight to marinate

COOK TIME: 2 hours 30 minutes

2 tablespoons extra-virgin olive oil

6 flanken-style grassfed short ribs, bones in, cut 2-inches thick (about 4 pounds)

1 tablespoon salt

1 tablespoon freshly ground black pepper

1 large onion, chopped

2 carrots, sliced

3 celery stalks, sliced

3 garlic cloves, sliced

40 ounces bone broth, divided

4 thyme sprigs

1. In a large sauté pan over medium heat, heat the oil. Season the ribs with the salt and pepper. Add them to the pan and cook turning once, until browned, about 10 minutes. Transfer the ribs to a large storage container with a lid and place them in a single layer. Leave the container uncovered.

2. Add the onion, carrots, celery, and garlic to the pan and cook over low heat, stirring occasionally until softened, about 10 minutes. Pour 20 ounces of broth into the pan and warm it through. Pour the mixture over the ribs and let cool. Cover and refrigerate overnight, turning the ribs once.

3. Preheat the oven to 350°F.

4. Transfer the short ribs and marinade to a large enameled Dutch oven. Add the remaining 20 ounces of bone broth and bring to a boil. Cover and braise in the lower third of the oven for 90 minutes, until the meat is tender but not falling apart.

5. Uncover and cook for 45 minutes more, turning the ribs once or twice, until the sauce is reduced by about half and the meat is very tender.

6. Transfer the meat to a clean, shallow baking dish, discarding the bones as they fall off. Strain the sauce into a heat-proof measuring cup and skim off as much fat as possible. Pour the sauce over the meat; there should be about 2 cups.

7. Preheat the broiler. Broil the meat, turning once or twice, until glazed and sizzling, about 10 minutes. Transfer the meat to plates, spoon the sauce on top, garnish with the thyme, and serve.

SERVING TIP: This is delicious when served with Parsnip Purée (page 63).

PER SERVING: CALORIES: 349; CARBS: 6G; SUGAR: 2G; FIBER: 2G; FAT: 20G; SATURATED FAT: 8; PROTEIN: 35G; SODIUM: 1255MG

curried cauliflower

DAIRY FREE • GLUTEN FREE • PALEO • QUICK & EASY

MAKES 4 TO 6 SERVINGS If you love curry, you'll love this dish! The combination of both beef and pork helps round out the flavors of this recipe.

PREP TIME: 10 minutes
COOK TIME: 20 minutes

1 onion, diced

1 garlic clove, sliced

1 tablespoon coconut oil

½ pound ground grassfed beef

½ pound ground pastured pork

1 teaspoon salt

1 red bell pepper, seeded and julienned

1 orange bell pepper, seeded and julienned

1 cup bite-size broccoli florets

1 cup coconut milk

10 ounces bone broth

1 (14-ounce) jar green curry paste

½ cup basil leaves, chopped

4 cups Cauliflower Rice (page 59)

1. In a large sauté pan over medium heat, sauté the onion and garlic in the oil for 3 minutes, stirring frequently.

2. Add the ground beef, ground pork, and salt to the pan. Break the meat into chunks with a large spoon. Cook until browned.

3. Remove the beef and pork mixture and set aside. Add the red and orange bell peppers and broccoli to the pan. Cook for 5 minutes.

4. Return the beef and pork mixture to the pan. Then add the coconut milk, broth, and green curry paste. Cook for 5 minutes. Stir in the basil leaves.

5. To serve, pour the curry over the cauliflower rice.

PER SERVING: CALORIES: 518; CARBS: 23G; SUGAR: 9G; FIBER: 7G; FAT: 31G; SATURATED FAT: 22G; PROTEIN: 28G; SODIUM: 1863MG

roasted chicken thighs

DAIRY FREE • PALEO

MAKES 4 TO 6 SERVINGS If I could only eat one part of a chicken, it would be the thighs, hands down! They are moist, tender, and covered with delicious crispy skin. This recipe honors the chicken thigh by keeping it simple yet delicious.

PREP TIME: 10 minutes, plus 1 hour to marinate
COOK TIME: 45 minutes

12 chicken thighs, bone in, skin on
¼ cup extra-virgin olive oil
¼ cup Chicken Bone Broth (page 30)
Juice of ½ lemon
1 tablespoon fresh rosemary leaves
1 tablespoon fresh thyme leaves
1 teaspoon garlic powder
1 teaspoon fish sauce
1 teaspoon salt

1. In a large bowl, combine all the ingredients to marinate the chicken thighs for a minimum of 1 hour.

2. Preheat the oven to 425°F. Line a deep roasting pan with aluminum foil and place the chicken thighs in a single layer in the pan.

3. Cook for 35 to 45 minutes, or until the internal temperature of the thighs reaches 170°F.

> **BONE BROTH-FRIENDLY TIP:** Keep leftover bones for your chicken bone broth. More bang for your buck!

PER SERVING: CALORIES: 588; CARBS: 1G; SUGAR: 0G; FIBER: 0G; FAT: 43G; SATURATED FAT: 10G; PROTEIN: 48G; SODIUM: 863MG

tuna stuffed peppers

DAIRY FREE • GLUTEN FREE • PALEO

MAKES 4 SERVINGS **Albacore tuna works perfectly in this dish as a stuffing for bell peppers. Instead of mayonnaise, I use avocados to bind the tuna mixture together. The fresh crunch of the jalapeño peppers adds heat and texture.**

PREP TIME: 10 minutes
COOK TIME: 25 minutes

4 large bell peppers
2 (5-ounce) cans albacore tuna
1 small onion, finely diced
1 small jalapeño pepper, finely diced
1 teaspoon freshly squeezed lemon juice
¼ cup bone broth
2 avocados
½ cup frozen peas
1 teaspoon salt
1 teaspoon freshly ground black pepper

1. Preheat the oven to 375°F.

2. On a clean cutting board, cut the top off each bell pepper. Scrape out any seeds.

3. Drain both cans of tuna. In a large mixing bowl, combine the tuna, onion, jalapeño, lemon juice, broth, avocados, peas, salt, and pepper. Mix well.

4. Stuff each bell pepper with ¼ of the mixture. Place on a baking sheet.

5. Cook for 25 minutes, or until the bell peppers are soft.

6. Let sit for 5 minutes before serving.

PER SERVING: CALORIES: 285; CARBS: 21G; SUGAR: 5G; FIBER: 9G; FAT: 14G; SATURATED FAT: 2G; PROTEIN: 21G; SODIUM: 820MG

spicy pineapple pork stir-fry

DAIRY FREE • PALEO

MAKES 4 SERVINGS The first time I made a stir-fry was with my grandfather when I was 10 years old. He showed me how to slice the peppers and thicken the sauce. This recipe is a spinoff of the traditional stir-fry I used to make with him, combining the sweetness of pineapples and the heat of Spicy Pork Bone Broth (page 34). It's a winning combination!

PREP TIME: 10 minutes

COOK TIME: 25 minutes

1 large onion, cut into ½-inch strips

2 garlic cloves, sliced

2 tablespoons coconut oil

4 boneless pastured pork chops, cut into ½-inch strips

2 large bell peppers, seeded and cut into ½-inch strips

1 serrano pepper, seeded and cut into ½-inch strips (optional)

1 cup broccoli florets

10 ounces Spicy Pork Bone Broth (page 34)

1 (14-ounce) can pineapple chunks (reserve liquid)

1 tablespoon coconut aminos

1 teaspoon fish sauce

1 teaspoon ground ginger

4 cups Cauliflower Rice (page 59)

1. In a large sauté pan over medium heat, sauté the onion and garlic in the oil for 3 minutes, stirring frequently.

2. Add the pork. Cook for 5 minutes, or until browned. Add the bell peppers, serrano (if using), and broccoli. Cook for 5 minutes, stirring frequently.

3. Add broth, pineapple chunks, coconut aminos, fish sauce, and ginger. Mix well and reduce the heat to medium-low. Add ¼ cup of pineapple juice from the can. Cook for 10 minutes.

4. Serve over cauliflower rice. Enjoy!

PER SERVING: CALORIES: 334; CARBS: 26G; SUGAR: 17G; FIBER: 6G; FAT: 13G; SATURATED FAT: 9G; PROTEIN: 28G; SODIUM: 477MG

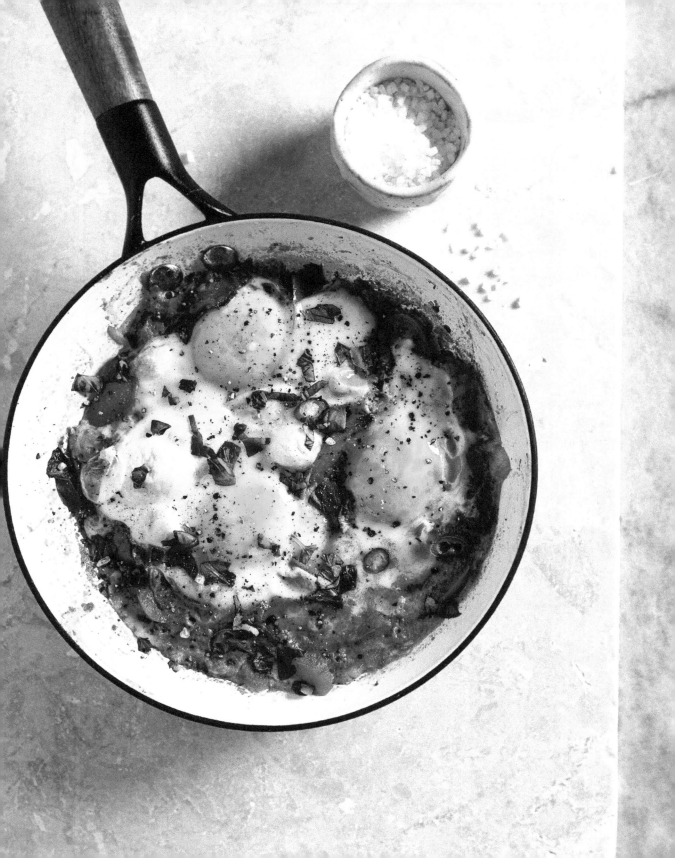

shakshuka

DAIRY FREE • GLUTEN FREE • PALEO

MAKES 5 SERVINGS Otherwise known as "eggs in purgatory," shakshuka, another North African dish, is great for breakfast. Let's be honest though, it's good any time of day. Add sautéed mushrooms for even more superfood properties.

PREP TIME: 5 minutes

COOK TIME: 40 minutes

10 cups chopped tomatoes

1 onion, chopped

4 garlic cloves, sliced

1 teaspoon salt

1 teaspoon red pepper flakes

10 ounces Beef Bone Broth (page 32)

5 eggs

1. In a medium saucepan over medium heat, combine the tomatoes, onion, garlic, salt, red pepper flakes, and broth. Cover and cook for 30 minutes, stirring often.

2. Mash the mixture with a potato masher until slightly chunky. Transfer to a sauté pan over medium heat and warm until bubbles begin to form on the surface.

3. Crack the eggs on top of the sauce, giving each egg room to cook individually, and cook for about 10 minutes until done to your liking.

ADD IN: Add some extra homemade sausage from the Red Pepper and Kale with Sausage over Spaghetti Squash recipe (page 132) to add some wonderful flavor and protein to the dish.

PER SERVING: CALORIES: 169; CARBS: 20G; SUGAR: 1G; FIBER: 4G; FAT: 6G; SATURATED FAT: 2G; PROTEIN: 12G; SODIUM: 570MG

red pepper and kale
with sausage over spaghetti squash

DAIRY FREE • GLUTEN FREE • PALEO

MAKES 6 SERVINGS The closest you'll get to spaghetti while on the 7-day bone broth diet is using spaghetti squash in place of noodles. The homemade sausage can be used in any dish, but pairs really well with the "spaghetti" in this dish.

PREP TIME: 10 minutes
COOK TIME: 55 minutes

FOR THE SAUSAGE

2 pounds ground pastured pork

1 teaspoon salt

1 teaspoon freshly ground black pepper

1 teaspoon dried parsley

1 teaspoon garlic powder

1 teaspoon onion powder

1 teaspoon paprika

¼ teaspoon red pepper flakes

½ teaspoon fennel seed

1 teaspoon dried thyme

FOR THE MAIN DISH

1 spaghetti squash, halved

1 tablespoon extra-virgin olive oil

1 onion, diced

1 red bell pepper, seeded and sliced

1 bunch kale, stemmed and chopped

10 ounces Spicy Pork Bone Broth (page 34)

TO MAKE THE SAUSAGE

In a large bowl, mix all the sausage ingredients together and set aside.

TO MAKE THE MAIN DISH

1. Preheat the oven to 375°F.

2. In a roasting pan, lay the spaghetti squash halves cut-side up and drizzle with the oil. Roast for 30 to 40 minutes.

3. Meanwhile, in a medium sauté pan over medium heat, sauté the onion, red pepper, and sausage mixture for 10 minutes, stirring frequently and chopping up the sausage as it cooks.

4. Add the kale and broth. Cook for 5 minutes, stirring frequently.

5. Use a fork to shred the squash into pasta-like strands. Divide evenly between bowls and top with the sausage mixture.

ADD IN: For extra heat, increase the red pepper flakes to ½ teaspoon.

PER SERVING: CALORIES: 480; CARBS: 13G; SUGAR: 4G; FIBER: 3G; FAT: 35G; SATURATED FAT: 12G; PROTEIN: 29G; SODIUM: 502MG

moroccan chicken tagine with apricots

DAIRY FREE • GLUTEN FREE • PALEO

MAKES 4 TO 6 SERVINGS **This North African–inspired recipe has a unique flavor profile. It is pleasing to the palate, making it perfect for dinner any night of the week.**

PREP TIME: 10 minutes, plus 30 minutes to marinate

COOK TIME: 45 minutes

6 chicken thighs, bone in, skin on

1 tablespoon extra-virgin olive oil

1 teaspoon salt

2 tablespoons coconut oil

1 onion, diced

2 garlic cloves, sliced

1 teaspoon ground cumin

1 teaspoon ground coriander

½ teaspoon ground cinnamon

½ teaspoon ground ginger

¼ teaspoon freshly ground black pepper

¼ teaspoon turmeric

⅛ teaspoon ground cloves

20 ounces Chicken Bone Broth (page 30)

½ cup dried apricots, sliced

1. In a medium bowl, marinate the chicken thighs in the olive oil and salt for 30 minutes.

2. In a nonstick sauté pan over medium-high heat, place the chicken thighs skin-side down in the coconut oil and sear for 5 minutes per side. Set aside.

3. Add the onion and garlic to the pan and cook for 5 minutes, stirring frequently.

4. Add the cumin, coriander, cinnamon, ginger, pepper, turmeric, and cloves. Cook for 3 minutes, stirring frequently.

5. Add the broth and stir to combine.

6. Return the chicken thighs to the pan, add the apricots, bring to a boil, then reduce the heat to low. Cover the pan and simmer for 30 minutes, or until the chicken is fully cooked. Enjoy!

PER SERVING: CALORIES: 404; CARBS: 13G; SUGAR: 10G; FIBER: 2G; FAT: 26G; SATURATED FAT: 11G; PROTEIN: 30G; SODIUM: 718MG

thai cashew zoodles

DAIRY FREE • GLUTEN FREE • PALEO

MAKES 6 SERVINGS **Even though this contains only vegetables, nuts, and seasonings, it is a fairly heavy dish. I was surprised how quickly this filled me up, leaving plenty of tasty Thai flavored zoodles for lunch the next day.**

PREP TIME: 10 minutes
COOK TIME: 15 minutes

20 ounces Spicy Pork Bone Broth (page 34)
2 bell peppers, seeded and cut into ½-inch-by-1-inch slices
2 cups spiralized butternut squash, divided
¼ cup cashew butter
¼ cup tahini
2 tablespoons coconut aminos
2 tablespoons freshly squeezed lime juice
2 teaspoons toasted sesame oil
¼ cup full-fat coconut milk
2 tablespoons toasted sesame seeds
1 cup fresh basil, chopped
½ cup fresh cilantro, chopped
1 cup cherry tomatoes, halved
1 teaspoon red pepper flakes
1 cup broccoli florets
½ cup roasted unsalted cashews

1. In a large pot over medium heat, bring the broth to a simmer. Add the bell peppers and 1 cup of butternut squash zoodles. Simmer for 5 minutes, or until the bell peppers soften but are still slightly al dente.

2. Meanwhile, mix the cashew butter and tahini together. When blended well, add the coconut aminos, lime juice, sesame oil, and coconut milk, and combine thoroughly. Then stir in the sesame seeds, basil, cilantro, tomatoes, and red pepper flakes. Set aside.

3. Transfer the cooked bell peppers and butternut squash to a serving bowl. Pour 1 cup of the bone broth liquid over the vegetables.

4. In the remaining broth in the large pot, simmer the broccoli and the remaining 1 cup of uncooked butternut zoodles for 3 minutes, until softened but still slightly al dente.

5. Transfer the broccoli and zoodles to the serving bowl. Stir to combine. Add the cashew butter and tahini mixture to the bowl. Mix until combined and top with the chopped cashews.

PER SERVING: CALORIES: 277; CARBS: 19G; SUGAR: 3G; FIBER: 5G; FAT: 19G; SATURATED FAT: 4G; PROTEIN: 12G; SODIUM: 137MG

roasted spatchcocked chicken

DAIRY FREE • GLUTEN FREE • PALEO

MAKES 4 SERVINGS Who doesn't love the smell of chicken roasting in the oven? Spatchcocking the bird—a method in which you cut poultry so it is nearly flat—quickens the cook time so you can get an entire chicken on your table in less than an hour. I love using the leftover bones from the chicken for my bone broth later on in the week.

PREP TIME: 10 minutes

COOK TIME: 45 minutes

1 (4-pound) pastured chicken

2 tablespoons coconut oil

¼ cup Chicken Bone Broth (page 30)

1 teaspoon salt

1 teaspoon freshly ground black pepper

1 lemon, halved

1 onion, sliced

1 teaspoon fresh thyme leaves

1. Preheat the oven to 425°F.

2. On a washable cutting board, place the chicken breast-side down. Starting at the thigh end, cut along the right side of the spine with kitchen shears. Turn the chicken around and cut along the left side of the spine. Flip the chicken and firmly press on the breastbone until flattened. Reserve the spine to make bone broth later.

3. In a small bowl, mix the oil, broth, salt, pepper, and juice of half a lemon. Mix until well combined. Spread the mixture over the chicken. Slice the remaining lemon half into slices, then place the slices under the chicken skin by gently separating the skin from the meat with your fingers.

4. Place the onion slices in a roasting pan and set the chicken on top. Sprinkle with the thyme. Roast for 45 minutes, or until the chicken reaches an internal temperature of 165°F.

5. Discard the lemon slices and carve the chicken into pieces, reserving the leftover bones and meat for making bone broth.

PER SERVING: CALORIES: 297; CARBS: 7G; SUGAR: 3G; FIBER: 2G; FAT: 22G; SATURATED FAT: 11G; PROTEIN: 22G; SODIUM: 1242MG

tomato smothered spaghetti squash with chicken fingers

GLUTEN FREE • PALEO

MAKES 4 SERVINGS If you're craving comfort food, you'll love this recipe. The homemade chicken fingers are delicious! Perfect for feeding your own kids or the kid in you.

PREP TIME: 10 minutes, plus 30 minutes to marinate

COOK TIME: 35 minutes

2 pounds boneless, skinless pastured chicken breast or thighs, cut into strips

¼ cup extra-virgin olive oil, plus more for drizzling

½ teaspoon salt

2 tablespoons bone broth

1 spaghetti squash, halved

1 cup cassava flour

½ teaspoon salt

½ teaspoon freshly ground black pepper

½ teaspoon garlic powder

½ teaspoon onion powder

¼ teaspoon cayenne pepper

¼ teaspoon paprika

¼ teaspoon turmeric

4 tablespoons ghee

Tomato sauce from Shakshuka (page 131) without the eggs, or 1 jar organic sauce

1. In a large bowl, combine the chicken, oil, salt, and broth. Marinate the chicken for 30 minutes.

2. Preheat the oven to 425°F.

3. In a roasting pan, lay the spaghetti squash halves, cut-side up, and drizzle with some oil. Roast for 30 minutes.

4. While the chicken is roasting, prepare the breading. In a medium bowl, combine the flour, salt, pepper, garlic powder, onion powder, cayenne, paprika, and turmeric.

5. When the squash is cooked remove it from the oven and let cool. Use a fork to shred the squash into pasta-like strands.

6. Dip the chicken strips into the breading. In a large sauté pan over medium-high heat, fry the chicken in the ghee for about 2 minutes per side, until lightly browned.

7. Warm the tomato sauce and pour it over the shredded spaghetti squash. Top with the chicken strips and serve.

PER SERVING: CALORIES: 857; CARBS: 59G; SUGAR: 14G; FIBER: 6G; FAT: 44G; SATURATED FAT: 14G; PROTEIN: 57G; SODIUM: 1395MG

roasted turkey

GLUTEN FREE • PALEO

MAKES 10 TO 12 SERVINGS Not just for Thanksgiving, this roasted turkey recipe is a great meal to rotate through your weekly lineup. The best part is that you can use the leftover bones for your Turkey Bone Broth (page 38). What a nice benefit!

PREP TIME: 10 minutes

COOK TIME: 2 hours 30 minutes

¼ cup ghee

¼ cup Turkey Bone Broth (page 38)

1 tablespoon sliced garlic, plus 1 teaspoon minced

2 lemons (1 sliced, 1 juiced)

10 thyme sprigs, plus 1 teaspoon leaves

1 (10-pound) fresh turkey

3 tablespoons salt

3 tablespoons freshly ground black pepper

1. Preheat the oven to 350°F.

2. In a small saucepan, combine the ghee, broth, 1 teaspoon of minced garlic, lemon juice, and 1 teaspoon of thyme leaves. Simmer for 5 minutes, stirring often. Set aside.

3. Remove all the innards from the turkey, rinse the bird with water, and dry thoroughly with paper towels. Liberally salt and pepper the turkey inside and out. Stuff the turkey cavity with the thyme sprigs, lemon slices, and 1 tablespoon of sliced garlic.

4. Brush the outside of the turkey with the bone broth mixture. Tie the legs together with string and tuck the wing tips under the body of the turkey.

5. Roast for 2½ hours or until the turkey reaches an internal temperature of 185°F. Every 30 minutes, baste the turkey with the pan juices.

6. Cover the turkey with aluminum foil and let cool for 20 minutes. Carve and enjoy!

> **BONE BROTH TIP:** Save the turkey carcass and any attached meat to make bone broth later.

PER SERVING: CALORIES: 417; CARBS: 1G; SUGAR: 0G; FIBER: 0G; FAT: 24G; SATURATED FAT: 9G; PROTEIN: 46G; SODIUM: 2226MG

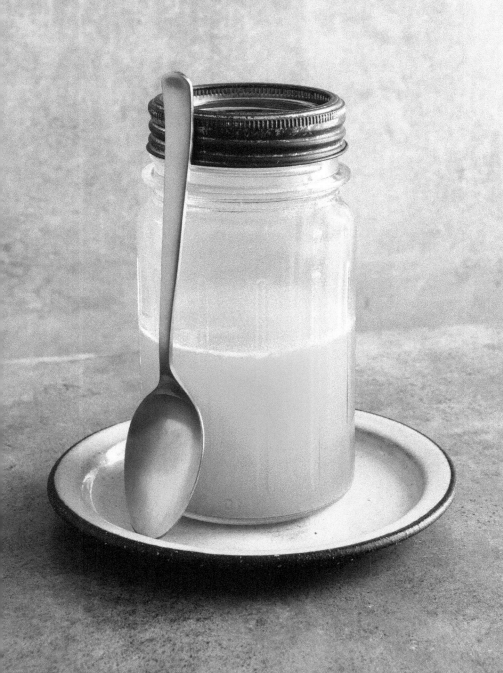

THE DIRTY DOZEN &
THE CLEAN FIFTEEN

A nonprofit and environmental watchdog organization called the Environmental Working Group (EWG) looks at data supplied by the US Department of Agriculture (USDA) and the Food and Drug Administration (FDA) about pesticide residues. Each year it compiles a list of the lowest and highest pesticide loads found in commercial crops. You can use these lists to decide which fruits and vegetables to buy organic to minimize your exposure to pesticides and which produce is considered safe enough to buy conventionally. This does not mean they are pesticide-free, though, so wash these fruits and vegetables thoroughly.

These lists change every year, so make sure you look up the most recent one before you fill your shopping cart. You'll find the most recent lists as well as a guide to pesticides in produce at EWG.org/FoodNews.

THE DIRTY DOZEN*

- Apples
- Celery
- Cherry tomatoes
- Cucumbers
- Grapes
- Nectarines (imported)
- Peaches
- Potatoes
- Snap peas (imported)
- Spinach
- Strawberries
- Sweet bell peppers

* Kale/Collard greens & Hot peppers

THE CLEAN FIFTEEN

- Asparagus
- Avocados
- Cabbage
- Cantaloupes (domestic)
- Cauliflower
- Eggplants
- Grapefruits
- Kiwis
- Mangos
- Onions
- Papayas
- Pineapples
- Sweet corn
- Sweet peas (frozen)
- Sweet potatoes

* In addition to the dirty dozen, the EWG added two produce contaminated with highly toxic organophosphate insecticides.

MEASUREMENT AND CONVERSION CHARTS

VOLUME EQUIVALENTS (LIQUID)

US STANDARD (OUNCES)	US STANDARD (APPROXIMATE)	METRIC
2 tablespoons	1 fl. oz.	30 mL
¼ cup	2 fl. oz.	60 mL
½ cup	4 fl. oz.	120 mL
1 cup	8 fl. oz.	240 mL
1½ cups	12 fl. oz	355 mL
2 cups or 1 pint	16 fl. oz.	475 mL
4 cups or 1 quart	32 fl. oz.	1 L
1 gallon	128 fl. oz.	4 L

OVEN TEMPERATURES

FAHRENHEIT (F)	CELSIUS (C) (APPROXIMATE)
250°F	120°C
300°F	150°C
325°F	165°C
350°F	180°C
375°F	190°C
400°F	200°C
425°F	220°C
450°F	230°C

VOLUME EQUIVALENTS (DRY)

US STANDARD	METRIC (APPROXIMATE)
⅛ teaspoon	0.5 mL
¼ teaspoon	1 mL
½ teaspoon	2 mL
¾ teaspoon	4 mL
1 teaspoon	5 mL
1 tablespoon	15 mL
¼ cup	59 mL
⅓ cup	79 mL
½ cup	118 mL
⅔ cup	156 mL
¾ cup	177 mL
1 cup	235 mL
2 cups or 1 pint	475 mL
3 cups	700 mL
4 cups or 1 quart	1 L

WEIGHT EQUIVALENTS

US STANDARD	METRIC (APPROXIMATE)
½ ounce	15 g
1 ounce	30 g
2 ounces	60 g
4 ounces	115 g
8 ounces	225 g
12 ounces	340 g
16 ounces or 1 pound	455 g

RESOURCES

COOKWARE

Cast-iron cookware (LeCreuset.com)

Chinois Mesh Strainer (New Star Food Service, Amazon.com)

Pressure Cooker (InstantPot.com)

FOOD

AGA Certified Grassfed & Finished Beef (Richard Family Ranch, www.richardsgrassfedbeef.com)

Bone Broth (Osso Good, www.ossogoodbones.com)

Celtic sea salt (www.selinanaturally.com)

Coconut oil (Dr. Bronner's)

Fish Sauce (Red Boat)

Ghee (4th and Heart, OMghee, Tin Star)

Grassfed Bison (The Honest Bison, www.thehonestbison.com)

Heritage, Pastured Turkey (Mary's Turkey, www.marysturkeys.com)

Pastured Chicken (Mary's Chicken, www.maryschickens.com)

Pastured Pork (Tara Firma Farms, www.tarafirmafarms.com)

Primal Palate (www.primalpalate.com)

REFERENCES

Acidic Body: A Body's Red Flag for Help. "Glycosaminoglycans (GAGs) depletion." http://acidicbody.com/glycosaminoglycans-gags-depletion.

Bensky, Dan, Steven Clavey, and Erich Stoger. *Chinese Herbal Medicine Materia Medica*. Seattle, WA: Eastland Press, 2004.

Damjanov, Ivan. *Pathology for the Health Professions*. St. Louis, MO: Elsevier Saunders, 2012.

Daniel, Kaayla. "Why Broth is Beautiful: Essential Roles for Proline, Glycine and Gelatin." The Weston A. Price Foundation. June 18, 2003. Accessed October 1, 2017. https://www.westonaprice.org/health-topics/why-broth-is-beautiful-essential-roles -for-proline-glycine-and-gelatin.

Dr. Axe: Food Is Medicine. "Bone Broth Benefits for Digestion, Arthritis and Cellulite." Accessed October 2, 2017. https://draxe.com/the-healing-power-of-bone-broth-for -digestion-arthritis-and-cellulite.

Gotthoffer, Nathan Ralph. *Gelatin in Nutrition and Medicine*. Grayslake IL: Great Lakes Gelatin Company, 2012.

Hampton, Tracy. "Organoids Reveal Clues to Gut-Brain Communication." *Jama* 318, no. 9 (September 2017): 787–8. doi:10.1001/jama.2017.11545.

Helander, H. F., and L. Fändriks. "Surface Area of the Digestive Tract—Revisited." *Scandinavian Journal of Gastroenterology* 49, no. 6 (June 2014): 681–9. doi:10.3109/0036 5521.2014.898326.

Kesser, Chris. "Bountiful Benefits of Bone Broth: a Comprehensive Guide." February 21, 2017. Accessed October 1, 2017. https://chriskresser.com/the-bountiful-benefits -of-bone-broth-a-comprehensive-guide.

Koyama, Y., A. Hirota, H. Mori, H. Takahara, K. Kuwaba, M. Kusubata, Y. Matsubara, S. Kasugai, M. Itoh, and S. Irie. "Ingestion of Gelatin has Differential Effect on Bone Mineral Density and Body Weight in Protein Undernutrition." *Journal of Nutritional Science and Vitaminology* 47, no. 1 (February 2001): 84–86.

Maciocia, G. *The Foundations of Chinese Medicine: A Comprehensive Text for Acupuncturists and Herbalists*. Edinburgh: Churchill Livingstone, 1989.

Mercola, Joseph. "Bone Broth—A Most Nourishing Food for Virtually Any Ailment." Mercola: Take Control of Your Health. Accessed October 2, 2017. https://articles. mercola.com/sites/articles/archive/2014/11/23/nourishing-bone-broth.aspx.

Morell, Sally Fallon and Kaayla T. Daniel. *Nourishing Broth: An Old-Fashioned Remedy for the Modern World*. New York, NY: Grand Central Life & Style, 2014.

Nichols, Hannah. "All You Need to Know about Bone Marrow." Medical News Today. Updated December 15, 2017. https://www.medicalnewstoday.com/articles/285666.php.

Petrucci, Kellyann. "My Secret to Anti-Aging, Weight Loss & Gut Health." Accessed October 2, 2017. https://www.mindbodygreen.com/0-22871/my-secret-to-antiaging -weight-loss-gut-health.html.

Tierra, Michael. *The Way of Herbs*. New York, NY: Pocket Books, 1998.

Unschuld, Paul U. *Medicine in China: A History of Ideas,* 25th Anniversary Edition. Los Angeles, CA: University of California Press, 2010.

RECIPE INDEX

INDEX

ACKNOWLEDGMENTS

I want to thank all of those who have poured their soul into researching preventive health and food as medicine. It is because of your work that we have gone on to study on our own and to add to it what we can. To my team at Osso Good. My partners, Jazz and Toran, who have helped me create a business that not only creates a high-quality bone broth, but also a business based on helping others. To Greg Willsey and Jill Costelow, who continually pour their heart and soul into making our dreams a reality. To the team at Osso Good who has become family, and the many others who have helped us succeed.

To my family for being my rock. Jazz, it isn't always easy, but with you by my side we can move mountains, one millimeter at a time. Mom and Dad Cochran, for giving me the world and letting me explore it to find my passions. But most of all, for instilling a love, passion, and dedication to the humble work we do day in and day out. Mom and Dad Hilmer, for always being there to lend an ear when we need it the most and for making family your number one priority. Melissa and Jessica, we may have been forced into sisterhood, but we have chosen to be best friends. To my family and dear friends, for your continued support, love, guidance, and example. Toran and Laura, Dane and Ann, Curtis and Noelle, Dave and Mary Claire, and Suzanne. And to all of those who continue to show support day in and day out. You know who you are.

To my team at Callisto, for helping put my thoughts into words and my words into a story.

Last but not least, I want to thank you for supporting our mission to bring slow-cooked, healing, and nourishing foods to a fast-paced world. "Be the change you wish to see in the world."

CPSIA information can be obtained
at www.ICGtesting.com
Printed in the USA
BVHW06s2250200518
516666BV00003B/3/P

9 781623 159986